Concise Guide to
Medications, Herbs and Supplements for the Horse

Also by David W. Ramey, DVM

The Anatomy of a Horse
Concise Guide to Arthritis in the Horse
Concise Guide to Colic in the Horse
Concise Guide to Laminitis in the Horse
Concise Guide to Medications and Supplements for the Horse
Concise Guide to Navicular Syndrome in the Horse
Concise Guide to Nutrition in the Horse
Concise Guide to Respiratory Disease in the Horse
Concise Guide to Tendon and Ligament Injuries in the Horse
A Consumer's Guide to Alternative Therapies in the Horse
Horsefeathers: Fact vs. Myths about Your Horse's Health

Concise Guide to
Medications, Herbs and Supplements for the Horse

David W. Ramey, DVM

TRAFALGAR SQUARE BOOKS
North Pomfret, Vermont

First published in 2007 by
Trafalgar Square Books
North Pomfret, Vermont 05053

Printed in the United States of America

Library of Congress Cataloging-in-Publication Data

Ramey, David W.
  A concise guide to medication, herbs, and supplements for the horse / David W. Ramey.
     p. cm.
  Rev. ed. of: Concise guide to medications & supplements for the horse. 1996.
  Includes bibliographical references and index.
  ISBN-13: 978-1-57076-365-6 (pbk.)
  ISBN-10: 1-57076-365-8 (pbk.)
  1. Horses--Diseases--Chemotherapy. 2. Horses--Feeding and feeds. 3. Veterinary drugs. 4. Feed additives. I. Ramey, David W. Concise guide to medications & supplements for the horse. II. Title.
  SF951.R23 2007
  636.1'0893--dc22
                                          2006033977

Book and cover design by Heather Mansfield
Typeface: Leawood and Sabon

10 9 8 7 6 5 4 3 2 1

CONTENTS

ACKNOWLEDGMENTS

I am thrilled that Trafalgar Square Books has decided to reissue this book, which was something of a landmark when it came out, and which proved to be very popular. Thanks especially to Martha Cook and to Caroline Robbins, who continue to support the idea that educating people who own horses is a good thing. Thanks also to all of my clients, who continue to comb the Internet and pepper me with questions about the lastest therapeutic trend. Thank you to Dr. Valerie Devaney, a defender of science, an advocate for horses, and as caring and thoughtful a veterinarian as could ever be, who was kind enough to read the entire book and suggest additions, point out errors and highlight areas that could be more clear. To my boys, Jackson and Aidan, watching you grow, win tournaments and belts, and hearing you continue to suggest—at least sometimes—that you think a veterinary career might not be all bad, is a constant source of wonder and wonderfulness. Finally, to Oryla, my wife, thanks for your support and love. Life's better with a real partner.

INTRODUCTION

The horse is a surprisingly sturdy creature and a marvel of engineering. He is a large system, one that possesses tremendous strength and endurance, but one that is able to function on just vegetable material and water. Left to their own devices, horses do pretty well.

Of course, horses are not left to their own devices. Once man found out that horses made great work animals, play partners and companions, it was inevitable that things would begin to happen to the horse. Man seems to have a peculiar inability to leave well enough alone. "Good enough," rarely is. What this means for horses is that people who own them want to help them to be the best that they can be (sometimes maybe even better than they can be).

In most cases, this desire to help the horse is a good thing. For example, when your horse has an infection, helping him by giving him antibiotics to kill the infection is a fairly straightforward concept.

There is a difference, however, between helping a horse get back to what he was and trying to make a horse be better than what he is. In an attempt to do the latter, many things are done to or given to horses to enhance performance, increase efficiency (whatever that means) or merely improve their appearance.

For example, a wide variety of nutrients can be demonstrated to be necessary in the normal diet of the horse. However, just because *some* of something is good does not mean that *more* of that same thing is necessarily better. For instance, iron is unquestionably needed by the horse for normal red blood cell formation. But more iron than what's required by the horse doesn't actually cause more red blood cells to be produced; in fact, too much iron can be toxic.

Frequently, the things that people do to "improve" their horses involve giving or applying one of a variety of medications and supplements that are marketed to the horse owner "over-the-counter." Most of these products are, fortunately, fairly benign. Many of them actually do what they claim to do (supply vitamins and minerals, for example). However, many of the claims made by the manufacturers of medications and supplements are so vague and general that it's difficult to figure out what, if anything, they are supposed to do.

The equine health pond has been made even murkier by the addition of various herbal products. These substances claim to be able to prevent and treat a bewildering array of equine problems (some of which may even exist). However, the field is full of claims and virtually bereft of evidence, and the use of herbs themselves poses some considerable questions, which, hopefully, this book will help clarify.

For the purposes of this book, a *drug* is defined as a substance that is used in the diagnosis, treatment or prevention of a disease. These substances are recognized and defined by the United States Food, Drug and Cosmetic Act. Their effects have been studied and their levels in blood and various tissues have been measured by scientists. Importantly, if a drug is given to an animal, its effect is usually predictable and controllable. Drugs are most commonly obtained by prescription or from your veterinarian. Therefore, their distribution and use is (ideally) controlled.

Herbs are like, and unlike, drugs. They are like drugs because if they work, it is due to active substances that have biological effects on the horse's body. They are unlike drugs in that they are largely unregulated and unstudied. They are not regulated for safety, for effectiveness or for purity. However, they are often advertised as if they are benign: "natural." The term natural is used to imply that herbs are harmless or have no undesired effects. That's not what natural means; both hurricanes and rattlesnakes are "natural." Of course, if a product doesn't have any effects then it isn't worth using, either.

Supplements, on the other hand, are a somewhat different ball game. Unlike most drugs, and some herbal remedies, supplements are not usually given because of disease. Instead, they are usually given to normal horses in an effort to "make up for" perceived deficiencies (real or imagined), to prevent various (bad) things from happening, or to make the horse somehow "better." Whether it be the composition of the hoof, the thickness of the hair or the overall sense of well-being that the horse is supposed to have, there are products out there that promise to help improve it. Supplements, at least those that are manufactured by large companies, would at least seem to be mostly safe for your horse.

However, there is generally little or no controlled data as to their effectiveness. It is important to note that supplements are not carefully studied, regulated or measured for their ability to do what the manufacturer says that they will do, or even regulated to contain what they say they contain.

There are many anecdotal reports about supplements, however. That is, there are stacks of testimonials—this trainer saying some supplement is great or that horse owner saying, "Thank you for your product!" Millions of dollars are spent by the horse-owning public on these products based on the allure of such testimony. Anecdotes and testimonials are wonderful, but they're simply stories of personal experiences (for which the trainer or owner may be compensated), and they are certainly no substitute for sound scientific investigation. While supplements are unlikely to hurt your horse, they may not help, either.

That being said, all you—the horse owner—really care about is doing the best that you can for your horse. Presumably, you will be somewhat curious about all the things you are going to be told that you should or must give to your horse. The purpose of this book is to help satisfy that curiosity. It is not intended to be a text on pharmacology (although some pharmacology is inevitable when dealing with the subject of drugs). This book is also not intended to be a catalogue of all the medications, supplements and herbal products available for the horse. That would be impossible, as new products seem to appear almost daily. Even a cursory review of this book, placed side-by-side with the first edition, would show numerous changes and additions. Still, by using this book to look for the ingredients listed on the product labels, you should be able to get an idea of what's in most of the products commonly used on horses and what those ingredients might actually do.

One other thing to remember: research is going on constantly. Companies develop and release products prior to a full investigation of their effects. Drugs, herbs and supplements may be safe for horses but may also be released for use prior to completely understanding what they do. In many cases, since there is so much new information, this means that there may be no consensus in the veterinary community as to the "right" or "best" way to use a particular medication. There may be many opinions as to "optimum" treatments and all of them may have some element of truth. Thus, you should rely on the experience of your veterinarian in selecting appropriate treatments for any condition of your horse that requires medical therapy.

This book is intended to help answer the cares and concerns of horse owners who are interested in many of the medications, supplements and botanical products available for their horses. It explains why these substances are given, how (or if) they work and whether they have significant side effects. You are going to find that there is information on product labels that conflicts with some of the information in this book. That's because while there's a seemingly endless variety of beneficial claims made for products sold for the horse (especially over-the-counter products), there's often little or no evidence to substantiate them. If you choose to take the manufacturer's claims at face value, remember: buyer beware.

Ideally, then, by reading this book, you will at least have some insight into the products that you may be advised to use to better your horse's health. That insight will help you make a more educated decision regarding your horse's health, and you will both be better for it.

Reader's Note

Please note that the drugs listed in the book are generally identified by their generic names in order to avoid having to list all the different products separately; likewise, the ingredients of various supplements should be looked for under the headings for their ingredients. Where the proprietary name for a drug is used commonly (such as Banamine®, which is a trademarked name that Schering-Plough Pharmaceuticals uses to market flunixin meglumine in the United States), the reader is usually referred to the generic heading. But to give you a hand in finding them, there is also an index of the brand names described in these pages at the end of the book.

Throughout the text, I often use the term "normal horse feed." Whenever I do source this as a general baseline, I'm simply referring to a diet high enough in calories for a specific animal. These calories can come from a variety of grains, legumes, concentrated feeds, or a combination of them.

CHAPTER

Medications, Herbs and Supplements for the Horse: An Overview

A lmost as important as which drug or product you give your horse is the route by which it is given. Drugs are most commonly given to the horse by one of three routes: *oral, intramuscular (IM)* or *intravenous (IV)*. A few drugs are applied to the surface of something; this is called *topical*, or *transdermal*, drug administration.

No route of administration is always "better" than another. Each route, however, has its own characteristic way of being absorbed into the horse's system. Each route has its own advantages.

Most drugs can only be given by one route; of course, there are exceptions. If given by a route other than that recommended, drugs that are otherwise safe can be dangerous. For example, the liquid preparation of phenylbutazone ("bute"), a commonly used anti-inflammatory agent, must be given intravenously. If it is given in the muscle, bute causes muscle irritation and abscesses because the solution is very irritating and acidic. Therefore, drugs should generally be given by the route recommended by the manufacturer (although your veterinarian may know of a safe alternative route for some drugs). Like most other things in life, you're generally better off if you follow the instructions.

INTRAVENOUS ADMINISTRATION
The *intravenous (IV)* route of administration puts a drug into the horse's system rapidly. It is generally used when a quick response is needed, such as in emergency situations or for inducing anesthesia or tranquilization. A drug given intravenously is rapidly diluted by the blood; this means that some irritating substances, or large volumes, can be given via the IV route but not by any other. When given in the vein, a drug also reaches a higher level in the system at

a more rapid rate than if it is given by one of the other routes. It is also removed from the system more rapidly when it is given IV. The preparations of a drug given intravenously must be *sterile* (free of contamination or microorganisms) to avoid a generalized infection in the horse receiving the drug.

Intravenous injections are most commonly given in the *jugular vein*, on the side of the horse's neck. Intravenous administration of a drug is not particularly difficult (once you know how) but it is important that it be done properly. Significant side effects can occur when an IV injection is done improperly. For example, if the injected substance is accidentally deposited outside of the jugular vein, infection, abscesses, swellings and soreness can occur. These problems from injection outside the vein can be serious enough in their own right; however, in addition, an even more serious and possibly permanent side effect, partial paralysis of the cartilage of the larynx *(roaring)*, can also result from a missed IV injection.

Here's why: in the back of the horse's mouth is the opening to the windpipe *(trachea)*. The opening is guarded by the two cartilages of the larynx, known as the *arytenoid cartilages*. Muscles attached to these cartilages pull them open, sort of like elevator doors, when the horse is breathing. The cartilages close when the horse swallows (this prevents food from going down into the lungs).

By some quirk of equine anatomy, the nerve that brings feeling and movement to the muscles of the cartilage on the left side of the larynx runs just alongside the left jugular vein, in a groove on the side of the horse's neck. By some quirk of human anatomy, most people are right-handed. Right-handers usually find it easier to make intravenous injections into the left jugular vein. If a substance is accidentally injected next to (instead of into) the vein, swelling and inflammation can result. The tissue irritation thus induced by the misplaced substance can envelop the nerve, often damaging or destroying it. Destruction of the nerve may result in a paralysis of the left arytenoid cartilage. (Incidentally, the nerves running to the right side of the larynx are different. Injection into the right jugular vein does not pose the same potential problems as does injection into the left vein.)

When a horse has left laryngeal paralysis, he frequently begins to make noise (roaring) when he exercises. This is because the paralysis prevents the airway from opening completely. Instead of opening up all the way, the paralyzed cartilage just hangs in the airway and vibrates (exactly like the paper in a kazoo). This is not dangerous to the horse but it can result in decreased performance.

An air passage obstructed by a paralyzed cartilage can reduce or stop the flow of air to the horse. Normal airway function is particularly important for racehorses. Racehorses need to have their airways completely open so they can get as much air into their lungs as possible when they are running at full speed. Show horses affected with a cartilage paralysis don't tend to have problems getting enough air to breathe because they don't exercise nearly as hard as racehorses; however, the loud noise they often make at exercise may be deemed undesirable.

Partial paralysis of the cartilages of the larynx generally does not get better on its own. The only treatment for the condition is surgery to "tie back" the paralyzed cartilage.

Another, even more serious complication of a misplaced intravenous injection again relates to the horse's anatomy. The jugular vein runs over the top of another important blood vessel, the *carotid artery*. The jugular vein carries blood to the heart. When a substance is given in the horse's vein, it has time to be diluted in the large volume of the horse's blood. The substance mixes in the blood as it passes through the horse's heart and lungs. Then the diluted substance is distributed to the rest of the body.

The carotid artery, however, carries blood from the heart directly to the horse's brain. If a drug is accidentally given into the carotid artery, it goes straight to the brain, minimally diluted. Direct delivery to the brain of a concentrated solution of a drug can knock a horse down to the ground or even kill him.

Obviously, then, it's important to be careful when giving an intravenous injection.

INTRAMUSCULAR DRUG ADMINISTRATION

Drugs given in the muscle are absorbed more slowly than those given in the vein. When a drug is given *intramuscularly (IM)*, the highest level of drug attained in the bloodstream is usually less than what can be reached by the intravenous route. However, levels for drugs given IM usually stay in the system for a longer time than those given IV. This can be an advantage in the treatment of some conditions.

Intramuscular injections are more easily given than IV injections, especially when the horse getting the shot is a bit fractious or unruly. Certain preparations, such as procaine penicillin, can only be given by IM injection. Like preparations for IV injection, IM products must also be sterile.

If you're not careful, it is possible to accidentally give an intravenous injection when intending to give an intramuscular one. When a needle is placed in the muscle, the end of it can come to rest inside a blood vessel (muscles are full of blood vessels). It is therefore important to pull back on the plonger of the syringe used to give the injection prior to depressing it. You want to make sure that you don't see any blood being sucked back into the syringe when you pull back on the plonger—this would indicate the needle is in a vein. Intramuscular drugs such as procaine penicillin can be dangerous—even deadly—if given intravenously.

Intramuscular injection is generally done directly into the large muscles of the neck or the big muscle groups of the hindquarters (other muscle groups can be used, but usually only with small volumes of watery solutions). The drug is then rapidly removed from the muscle by the horse's circulatory system. If a drug is accidentally given between muscle groups (in a fascial plane) it may not be well absorbed. Injection between muscles may also result in swellings or abscesses. It is therefore recommended that intramuscular injection not be given high up on the neck, toward the head. It is much easier to accidentally get a needle between the many groups of small muscles in that area than it is if the injection is given lower on the neck.

Inevitably, some horses develop abscesses or swellings from intramuscular injection. If an injection abscess forms, it tries to open to the outside of the horse and drain. (Abscesses always expand toward the area of least resistance—the skin—and in the direction of the pull of gravity.)

In anticipation of injection abscesses, IM injection into the muscles of the hip is generally not recommended in horses, even though the muscles there are large. If an abscess from injection happens on the hip, in the gluteal muscles, the abscess fluid can't travel up and out of the horse's body (away from the pull of gravity). Instead, gravity pulls the fluid down the leg (it "gravitates"). The abscess fluid must dissect its way all the way down through the muscle groups of the limb to get out, and it may not find a spot to exit until it reaches a point quite low on the leg. This can take a long time (up to several months), and in the meantime, the horse may be very sore and lame.

ORAL DRUG ADMINISTRATION

The *oral* route of drug administration has very little inherent risk associated with it, as long as the substances given aren't toxic. Blood levels of drugs given orally reach much the same levels as do drugs given by intramuscular injection. One of the nice things about drugs given orally is that they do not have to be sterile.

Even though oral drug administration is safe and effective, it is not necessarily easy. Since horses can be pretty discriminating eaters, attempting to give a drug orally by hiding it in the feed can be quite frustrating. No amount of molasses, honey or pancake syrup can kill the "bad" taste of some medication for finicky horses. These picky eaters are able to leave a neat little pile of medication in the feeder after they are finished eating the feed in which their medication was "hidden."

Consequently, a number of medications have been formulated into pastes that you deposit inside the horse's mouth. However, since horses can also be pretty fussy about having things put in their mouths, this isn't necessarily the answer, either. Paste medications can be squirted into (and sometimes spit right back out of) the horse's mouth. This same problem can be experienced when trying to give a horse a liquid medication or attempting to place pills in the back of his throat.

These are horses, after all! Even though there are a lot of *effective* ways to medicate a horse, sometimes there is no *easy* way.

TOPICAL AND/OR TRANSDERMAL ADMINISTRATION

A few medications are intended to be applied *topically*, that is, to surfaces of the horse rather than into the muscle, mouth or bloodstream. For example, medicated ointments or solutions are often applied topically onto healing wounds, or injured eyes, in hopes of controlling or preventing infection and/or inflammation. There are also topical ointments or creams that can be used in an effort to control surface cancers. Interestingly, inhaled medications used to control airway problems in horses are also considered a "topical" administration, because they directly affect the surface of the air passages of the lungs, with little effect on the horse's system.

Other medications are applied onto the skin, but may also have effects on deeper tissues. In these preparations, the medication is supposed to cross (*trans-*) the skin (*dermal*) and deliver its benefits to the structures below the skin.

Medication applied to the surface of the horse's body is usually convenient to use because it doesn't have to be sterile. Since most of them are easily applied (with the exception of inhaled medications in some horses), they also give eager horse owners something satisfying to do for their injured horse. On the downside, some of the medications applied to the horse's skin have the potential to be very irritating, so make sure you ask your veterinarian before you go rubbing some well-intentioned "goo" on your horse for days on end.

There's also some question as to how effective or necessary some topical medications really are. For example, the routine use of antibiotic ointments for the treatment of wounds that have been sutured closed seems questionable, as is the concept of topical preparations "drawing out" infections from hooves, jaws or other body parts (see Wound Treatments, p. 196, and Poultice, p. 157).

DRUG DOSAGE

It is always important to follow the recommended dosage schedule of any drug given to your horse. The *dosage schedule* is affected by a number of factors, including how rapidly the drug is removed from the system, what level of the drug needs to be maintained in the system for it to be effective and what effect is desired. For example, it may be desirable to have a horse more or less tranquilized, depending on what you want to do to the horse.

For drugs to be effective, their dosage schedules must be followed closely. A dosage schedule of "three times a day" is more properly stated as "every eight hours"; giving a three-times-a-day medication at eight o'clock in the morning, at noon and at six in the evening may result in drug levels that are too high at some times and non-existent at others. Making sure that your horse gets his drugs at the right time may require some dedication from you. Your veterinarian should advise you as to the proper dosage schedule for drugs.

In addition to the proper dosage interval, the proper dose of a drug should also be followed. Drugs are not dangerous; nor are they generally harmless. Drugs that are safe at one dose may be dangerous at twice the dose. For this reason, you should not automatically assume that, just because your horse is not getting better as quickly as you think he should, by increasing the dose you will help him get better faster (that is, the "bigger hammer" theory is rarely useful, except sometimes in hammering). More is *not* always better. In fact, when it comes to drugs and other effective substances, it may be toxic. In addition, doubling the dose of a drug does not necessarily increase its effectiveness. A doubled dose may not even dramatically increase the time that a particular dose will stay in the system. This is because of what is known as the *half-life* of the drug.

When a drug is put into the horse's system, it immediately begins to be removed as a result of the horse's normal metabolic functions. Pharmacologists measure the time it takes for half of the initial dose to be removed from the horse's system. This is called the half-life of the drug. It gives pharmacologists a useful measure of the length of time that a particular drug may be effective in the horse's system.

If you double the dose of a drug, you increase its duration in the system by one half-life. If the half-life of a particular drug is four hours, doubling the dose only increases the length of time that the drug is in the system by that much time. However, while doubling the dose of a drug may not significantly prolong the time that the drug is in the system, doubling the dose can significantly increase the potential for adverse side effects. Therefore, you should always check with your veterinarian before altering the dose of any prescribed drug from that which is recommended.

DRUG LABELING: LIMITATIONS AND APPLICATIONS

Not all drugs used in horses have been specifically tested on horses. Veterinarians have broad authority in prescribing drugs for horses. It is tremendously difficult to bring a drug to market through the morass of testing procedures required by the US Food and Drug Administration (USFDA). Each drug has to be tested for each species in which it is to be used and for each specific use for which a benefit is claimed. This can be extremely expensive for the drug companies. Thus, not all drugs that are used in horses have been specifically approved for use in them, nor are all the drugs given to horses used according to the label directions.

For example, the label directive "Not for use in horses intended for food" is put there so that companies don't have to test for drug residues in horses that may end up entering the food chain. Ditto the warning, "Not for pregnant mares." Rather than pay for the testing on specific animals, companies tell you not to use the drug on those horses in an untested category. Similarly, gentamycin sulfate, a commonly used antibiotic, is approved for use in the uterus of mares only. However, the drug is frequently given in the muscle to treat bacterial infection of various areas. The company that makes gentamycin didn't want to pay to test the drug for safety when administered in the muscle, so they put a restrictive label on it. Nonetheless, veterinarians have used gentamycin sulfate for years in a manner other than that which is directed on the label. It has been found to be safe and effective. Veterinarians have wide discretion in trying to make use of any drug available that can potentially help sick horses. They usually know what you can and cannot do. They are the ones to ask about drugs.

By and large, drugs are wonderfully safe and effective when prescribed appropriately. However, it's a fact that all drugs are also potentially toxic substances. Paracelsus (1493–1541) was a Swiss doctor who was the first to suggest that disease occurred as a result of some specific cause outside the body. He noted, "All substances are poisons, for there is nothing without poisonous qualities. It is only the dose which makes a substance poisonous." After correct diagnosis, and when given in the proper dosage and by recommended routes of administration, drugs are likely to produce beneficial effects. They should be used accordingly.

OVER-THE-COUNTER PRODUCTS

Equine health care is complicated by the fact that there are a tremendous number of *over-the-counter* products—which would essentially include every herbal product and supplement—sold to horse owners. Concerned horse owners are usually trying to make their horses "better," with or without the aid of professional veterinary care. Such efforts are roughly akin to prescribing home remedies for yourself (or your friends). If a problem is self-limiting, incurable or nonexistent (or if it only exists in the mind of the horse owner), such an approach is likely to work out fine as long as no harm is done. If, however, there's a real disease process to be fought, such an approach can prevent or delay effective treatments.

Sometimes, over-the-counter products *do* seem to work. For example, if you have a cold, most of the time you'll eventually be just fine no matter what treatment you prescribe for yourself. This is because the body has a tremendous capacity and urge to heal, and most problems do get better. But sometimes the medication or over-the-counter products get the credit for healing that would have occurred anyway. The old saying is apt: "If you take medicine for your cold, it'll go away in seven days, but if you don't treat it, it'll hang on for a week!" Of course, if you have a serious problem, such as pneumonia, over-the-counter products aren't likely to do much good in curing it.

Over-the-counter products for horses make a wide variety of claims as to their effectiveness. Their claims are, by necessity, very general and vague. If over-the-counter medications made specific claims about their effectiveness, they would be subject to the same rules and regulations that confront the manufacturers of pharmaceutical products. They would be regulated by the US Food and Drug Administration. Drug manufacturers have to go through a variety of steps to make sure that their products are safe and actually do what they claim to do. Plus, manufactured drugs have to meet quality manufacturing standards for purity. Therefore, the specific effects of many supplemental products are poorly understood, if they are understood at all.

HERBAL PRODUCTS

Herbal History
As far back as evidence can be gathered, humans used various plants to treat their ailments, and presumably, those of their animals. Prescriptions for the use of various plants can be found in the medical lexicon of virtually every society in recorded history. However, herbal medications lost popularity as they could no longer match the advances of science and the resulting public trust that accompanied

those advances. The trend from crude plant to synthetic drug has continued, but due to the obvious fact that some herbal and botanical remedies contain pharmacologically active ingredients, the development of drugs from plants continues, and many drug companies are engaged in large-scale pharmacological screening of herbs.

The history of veterinary applications of herbals and botanicals is long and well-documented. For example, black and white helle-bore (*Helleborus niger* and *Veratrum album*, respectively) was pierced through the ears of horses and sheep by Pliny in the first century A.D., as well as in the early twentieth century as a purgative, emetic, anthelmintic and parasiticide (although it caused death in many animals). Historical prescriptions for herbal use can be found in such diverse sources as the Chinese *Yuan Heng liaoma ji* and in the medicinal practices of the North American Indian. Botanical "horse medicines" were provided during the Civil War. Even as late as 1957, popular books continued to list such substances as aconite, belladonna, cinchone, ipecac, nux vomica (strychnine) and tobacco for veterinary use. However, more recently, such titles were in scant evidence—until the latest revival of interest in the use of herbal and botanical veterinary remedies.

The active ingredients of some pharmaceuticals are identical to, or derivatives of, bioactive constituents of historic folk remedies. Herbal and botanical sources form the origin of as much as 30 percent of all modern pharmaceuticals. For example, aspirin (acetylsalicylic acid) is a derivative of salicylic acid, which, as salicin (salicyl alcohol plus a sugar molecule), occurs in the flower buds of the meadowsweet (spirea) and in the bark and leaves of several trees, notably the white willow *(Salix alba)*. White-willow-bark extracts were used for centuries as a pain remedy. Quinine was an important anti-fever agent and was widely employed for the treatment of fever of virtually any origin.

However, the fact that herbal products were used throughout history may also overlook real problems. For example, in order to ingest one gram of salicin (the parent of salicylate drugs and only about half as potent as aspirin) from willow bark, one would have to ingest at least 14 grams of the bark. The tannins in willow bark, as well as salicin, are very irritating to the stomach, so consuming this much bark would likely give you quite a bellyache. Another significant problem is the natural variation in plants. Different species of the same plant may have active compounds of varying qualities. The potency of such compounds deteriorates at unknown rates. Different compounds have various absorption rates from the gastrointestinal tract and there are also variations from batch to batch, depending on growing conditions.

In addition, the current usage of botanicals is quite different from their historical use. Historically, herbs were used in small amounts as specific treatments (rather than prophylactically in order to *prevent* health problems); in crude form (as opposed to enriched extracts); and not in association with other synthetic medications (removing concerns about interactions between herbs and drugs). The indications for using a given botanical were poorly defined. Dosages were, unavoidably, arbitrary because the concentrations of the active ingredient were unknown. Any number of contaminants may have been present. True plant identities are doubtful, both in regard to genus and species. The transmission of information was haphazard; herbalists copied extensively from one another over millennia and mixed accurate (by modern standards) information with nonsense, misconceptions and inaccuracies. Most important, many remedies simply did not work, and some were harmful or even deadly, but society was far more willing to accept risk in the treatment of disease. Accordingly, it may not be possible to use the historical record as a guide for many of the currently advocated uses of herbal and botanical products.

The historical record is also rather sobering when it comes to considering the question of whether herbal and botanical products are effective medicine. Historically, herbal and botanical medicines were not responsible for any measurable improvement in human health. In 1900, life expectancy was 45 years; however, in 1996 it was 76.1 years. These dramatic changes were largely due to clean water, vaccination and the ability to control infection via pharmacology.

When discussing the historical efficacy of herbal medications, one must also ask the question, "Effective compared to what?" Medical treatments available during the time of wide herbal use—such as "bleeding" or prescribing large doses of mercury salts—were largely ineffective. The use of a botanical product that didn't kill a person immediately might therefore be expected to do more good than other therapies that were available at the time.

The nature of the claims made for efficacy and the vagueness of the conditions treated make it exceedingly difficult to objectively evaluate the true utility of the plant-based remedies employed throughout history. In the past, the emphasis for their use was on treatment of symptoms, rather than underlying disease conditions (which had yet to be identified), such as "liver malfunction" or "dropsy." Elimination of the symptom, rather than elimination of the underlying problem, was the criterion for treatment "success." For example, if a fever went away after ingesting willow bark, the treatment would have "worked," although the disease process that caused the fever might have continued on, unaffected by the treatment.

Herbs and Science

Today, in laboratory settings, plant extracts have been shown to have a variety of pharmacologic effects, including anti-inflammatory, vasodilatory, anti-microbial, anti-convulsant, sedative and anti-fever effects. This should not be surprising, as many plants contain pharmacologically active ingredients, some of which are highly toxic. These sorts of substances are thought to be defense mechanisms for survival of the plants—other species learned to avoid plants that caused irritation, illness or death. Whether the plants or extracts that have been shown to have pharmacologic effects can be safely or effectively used as medicine is another question, and one that largely has yet to be answered.

When one considers the available evidence on the use of herbal medicines in people, one might conclude that, as far as an individual product goes, it might be "promising." However, only very rarely is there convincing evidence, or evidence that is considered sufficient to make a sound clinical decision for prescribing them. Most studies, or reviews of studies, show that the reported effects of herbal products seem to be rather limited, or need further confirmation by well-designed trials, or both. In addition, data that directly compares herbal remedies with well-established pharmaceutical products is often not available or does not provide much useful information (for example, data may be derived from studies that failed to include a placebo group).

A basic problem concerning all clinical research in herbal medicines is the question of whether different products, extracts, or even different lots of the same extract are comparable and equivalent. For example, echinacea products may contain other plant extracts, different plant species, different parts of the plant (herb, root, both) and might have been produced in quite different manners. In addition, the concentration of active ingredients can vary dramatically depending on where the plants were grown or when they were harvested. Finally, even a claim of "standardization" does not mean the preparation is accurately labeled, nor does it indicate less variability in concentration of constituents of the herb—any given bottle of an herb may contain different amounts of an active substance than another bottle of the same herb.

Such inherent variation in products means that it may not be possible to extrapolate the results of any one study to any particular product. And, of course, almost all trials of individual herbal products have been done in people; applying the findings of individual trials in human medicine to animal patients' care is problematic because different species may react to the same substance in different ways.

Nevertheless, popular herbalism (with its slogan of "botanicals are safer") appears to have abandoned most of the obvious pharmacologically active herbs (such as belladonna, ergot and colchicum) to the pharmaceutical industry, since their therapeutic window is so narrow and misuse can be deadly. Those that remain in more common use are not likely to be either very potent or very toxic. Indeed, not only are popular herbal products not likely to be very potent or toxic, many of the products intended for use in horses contain ingredients with no recognized therapeutic value at all. That is, the products may contain a variety of plants, but the plants don't necessarily do anything other than take up space in the package. Herbs such as burdock root, "cleavers" (derived from a climbing plant that is common in England), oregano and dandelion have no currently known or demonstrated therapeutic value, although all of them are ingredients in an over-the-counter "anti-itch" preparation sold to horse owners.

Herbal products may be prescribed for reasons that diverge from known medical practice. That is, treatments may be prescribed or based on vague rationales for which there is no proof, or which make no sense. For example, observations such as, "underfunctioning of a patient's systems of elimination" or "an accumulation of metabolic waste products" make no medical sense whatsoever. However, based on such fanciful suppositions, plants with purported diuretic or laxative actions might then be prescribed. Herbal products might also be prescribed to "support" various body systems, even though the term "support" is vague and ill-defined, there may be no evidence that such systems are in need of support, and there may be no evidence that the prescribed plant supports the systems anyway!

Herbal Safety

That said, herbal medicines do present real risks of undesired side effects and interactions with genuine pharmaceuticals. Allergic reactions, toxic reactions, adverse effects related to an herb's desired pharmacological actions and possible mutagenic effects have been identified. Several reviews summarizing side effects and interactions have been published. For example, nonsteroidal anti-inflammatory drugs (NSAIDs) have the potential to interact with a number of herbal supplements that are known to possess activity against blood clotting. Given the lack of information about such interactions in horses, it is probably best to avoid giving drugs and herbal products at the same time.

Herbal products may also be contaminated, adulterated or misidentified. For example, in 1998, the California Department of Health reported that 32 percent of Asian patent medicines sold in that state contained undeclared pharmaceuticals or heavy metals; this appears to be a particular problem in herbal preparations from Asian sources. Outright fraud also exists: in 2003, the Australian Therapeutic Goods Administration (TGA) suspended the license held by Pan Pharmaceuticals Limited of Sydney to manufacture medicine because of serious concerns about the quality and safety of their product. Because of such problems, calls for tighter regulation of botanical medicines have appeared.

Controlled studies on the clinical effects of herbal or botanical preparations in horses are virtually nonexistent. It's usually not known how the doses are obtained; they are often "proportional" to those used in human herbal medicine. However, it should be kept in mind that experience with pharmaceuticals has shown that extrapolating dosage or toxicity data from one species to another can be dangerous. Due to their inherent toxicity, some herbal remedies should not be used under any circumstance. Others—such as tea tree oil—while generally safe at some strengths, can cause significant adverse effects at others. In addition, because some herbal remedies contain multiple, biologically active constituents, interaction with conventional drugs is also a concern.

SUPPLEMENTS

By definition, a supplement is something that is provided to complete something, to make up for a deficiency or to extend or strengthen the whole (*American Heritage Dictionary of the English Language*. 3rd ed. Boston: Houghton Mifflin Company, 1992). Supplements that are provided to the horse's diet purport to do most or all of these things.

Supplementing for "Deficiencies"

Almost without question, the most common deficiency seen in the horse is a lack of adequate calories in the diet. Calories supply the chemical energy needed for the horse to run his body. Work such as exercise, lactation or growth requires a lot of calories. As such, horses that work hard may need more feed than what is routinely given to them.

However, there is a big difference between the chemical energy supplied by calories, and the less tangible concept of "feeling energetic." It's this latter concept that many horse owners fret over, and because of such fretting, there are many supplements marketed to horse owners that claim to "help" the horse with perceived deficiencies in energy. Most of these contain a variety of vitamins, minerals or proteins.

If horses are calorie-deficient—lacking in enough fuel to run their bodies—they lose weight, are in poor condition and may not feel energetic. However, these issues are not helped by any amount of supplemental vitamins or minerals. Of course, in many horses, the problem is too many calories; under such circumstances, these horses get fat (as would anyone eating too much).

People being people, however, generally overlook insufficient feed as a cause of a lack of energy and weight loss in their horse. Finding out that your horse is losing weight because he's not getting enough to eat is sort of like finding out that your washing machine doesn't work because you forgot to plug it in. You're happy to find out what the problem is, but it's kind of embarrassing and you'd really rather it be something else.

In fact, horses are rarely deficient in anything besides energy. (There are some exceptions; for example, certain parts of the United States have soil that is deficient in the trace mineral selenium, and horses in these areas may benefit from selenium supplementation.) It is very difficult to create a diet of "normal" horse feed that supplies enough calories for a horse's systems to run but that is also deficient in protein, vitamins and minerals. Vitamins, minerals and protein all have important functions in the horse; however, providing more of any of these substances than what is needed for a particular function will not cause the horse to do that function better. Nor are vitamins and minerals necessarily benign. In fact, toxicities of vitamins and minerals have been reported in the horse (though rarely).

There is, of course, no way to measure a horse's "energy levels." In fact, it's likely that any effects of vitamin and mineral supplements intended to make horses feel more "energetic" are psychological, exerting their most significant effects on the minds of horse owners. One might suggest that so long as the owner is happy, then it doesn't really matter that the effect is purely psychological. That's fine, as long as you can afford it and don't mind contributing toward the wealth of supplement makers. Just be sure you aren't neglecting real problems while chasing some attractively packaged "fix."

Dietary protein supplements are also commonly given to horses by their well-meaning owners. Unquestionably, the horse needs protein to build body tissue, but they really don't need very much of it. Extra dietary protein taken in by the horse is *not* beneficial (nor is it harmful). Nor do protein requirements in horses go up when they exercise. Excess protein is merely digested by the horse and converted to energy. Protein supplements are mostly just relatively expensive sources of supplemental energy for the horse.

Supplementing to "Strengthen" the Horse

The other defined function of supplements is to complete or strengthen the whole (horse, in this case). In this regard, supplements are commonly turned to in efforts to "improve" the horse, or to make him "better," at least in the mind of the owner. This generally means that the owner wants the horse to be better than, or somehow different from the way he actually is (a problem that plagues many relationships).

Consequently, a variety of supplements are available that claim a mind-boggling array of beneficial effects. The linguistic legerdemain invoked in support of various supplements strains even the thickest thesaurus. The following is a list of claims that have been taken from advertisements for various feed supplements:

- "Improves overall bloom"
- "Improves disposition"
- "Better general health"
- "Lengthens attention span"
- "Increases mental stability"
- "Helps hyper horses come down and lackadaisical horses come up"
- "Significant improvement in comfort"
- "Improves digestion"
- "Supports joint health [kidney function, immune system, liver function, etc.]"
- "Boosts the immune system"
- "Eliminates toxins"

All of these claims are truly amazing. Unfortunately, they are almost totally meaningless. For example, a supplement may be promoted to "improve performance." In reality, since "performance" is such a vague concept and "improvement" is so subjective, such claims are difficult, if not impossible, to measure.

Some such claims are ridiculous. There are not "toxins" circulating in the horse's body that need to be removed, and there is no evidence that products that claim to do such have any effect whatsoever. The term "support," as applied to various systems, has no medical meaning. In addition, some of the claims may even be for things that you wouldn't want. For example, a "boosted" immune system isn't necessarily a good thing; allergies and autoimmune conditions are two diseases characterized by a "boosted" immune system ("boost" being a synonym for "greater than normal").

As was mentioned in the introduction of this book, if *specific* claims were made for supplements ("This product is proven effective for the relief of pain and inflammation associated with chronic arthritis," for example), they would fall under all the rules and regulations that the manufacturers of drugs are subject to. Supplement manufacturers would have to prove that their products actually work if they were held to these standards. Since supplement manufacturers don't want to be held to the same standards as the drug manufacturers, they usually don't make specific claims as to the effectiveness or method of action of their products.

Supplements are also promoted by stating the individual ingredients and how they are used in the horse. Then, either directly or by implication, the horse owner is led to believe that the horse may not be getting enough of that ingredient. For example, the statement "This supplement contains fourteen amino acids. If any one of them is deficient in the diet, the horse's protein needs will not be fulfilled" is undoubtedly true. However, protein or amino acid deficient diets are essentially never reported as problems in the horse. Thus, supplementation with amino acids is rarely, if ever, required. Similar examples can be given for vitamins, minerals and electrolytes, the other most commonly supplemented substances.

Indeed, supplementing to prevent a problem that is almost undoubtedly not going to occur—such as an amino acid deficiency—just doesn't make sense. Say, for example, someone tried to sell you a bottle of rhinoceros repellant to prevent a tragedy just in case an angry rhino came storming by your horse's stall. Unless you keep your horse in the middle of the African veldt, buying such a product isn't likely to be necessary, even if it could be shown to work. And, it would be awfully hard to prove such a product was effective under any circumstance—if you bought a bottle of "Rhinomore," and no rhinos visited your horse's stable in, say, suburban Connecticut, would that prove to you that the product "worked"?

PRODUCT LABELING

It is very important that you read the labels of supplements for your horse. You not only want to find out what the supplements are supposed to do, you should also determine what is in the supplements that is supposed to cause the beneficial effects. Some over-the-counter medications and supplements do not even supply a list of ingredients! It seems foolish, at best, to use a product on your horse that does not reveal its ingredients. After all, your horse is relying on you to take care of him. If products don't care enough to tell you what you are giving to your horse, why should you care to use them?

If the supplement or over-the-counter medication that you use for your horse has listed its ingredients, look for them under the various individual headings in this book. Then you can at least try to understand what, if any, beneficial effects can be expected.

CHAPTER

Medication and the Performance Horse

Horses find themselves in a variety of sporting competitions, such as racing, jumping, eventing, Western events and dressage. Horses are athletes. Like all athletes, some will be better at their particular sport than others. Of course, people are rarely willing to accept the inherent natural limitations of an individual animal. Not only that, but in competitions almost everyone seems to be looking for an "edge" to make their horses just a little better. Accordingly, they may try to influence the horse's performance through various medications.

MEDICATION TO INCREASE PERFORMANCE

In some horses, medication is given in hopes that the horse's performance will be improved beyond what it would be without the medication. Examples of such medication might be stimulants, such as amphetamines or narcotics, used in an effort to "fire up" racehorses. (Unlike their effects in people, narcotics tend to cause excitement in horses.) Similarly, vitamins or anabolic steroids are sometimes used in an attempt to make racehorses or show horses "stronger" or more aggressive.

The effectiveness of stimulant medication in improving horse performance is not at all clear. When a horse is racing, he is being asked for an all-out, maximum effort. The idea of giving stimulants, then, is to put something into the horse that will make him do *more* than that which he is ordinarily capable of doing with his maximum effort. Whether this can be done is certainly questionable; after all, the horse can only do what he can do. No studies have shown that stimulant drugs have any effect on improving the performance of racehorses.

"Jugs" of fluids and vitamins, or injections of vitamins such as cyanocobalamin (vitamin B$_{12}$) are commonly given to try to make horses more energetic or to increase their red blood cell count. However, the administration of vitamins before a race or a show certainly never has been shown to have any beneficial effect in horses. Treatments such as these have been consistently ineffective in causing any changes in horses that have received them. However, being somewhat expensive, these treatments do consistently make the horse owner somewhat poorer.

On the other hand, anabolic steroids, another class of drugs purported to increase performance, at least have the potential to do so. These drugs can increase muscle mass, which is why they are used illegally by human weight lifters, football players and track stars. However, one study done in Scotland failed to show any increase in performance in racehorses given these drugs and no studies have reported them to actually be beneficial for such a purpose.

Anabolic steroids do have *androgenic effects*; that is, they may make horses demonstrate aggressive, stallion-like behavior. For this reason, they are sometimes used in efforts to make horses that seem to lack energy more dynamic. Again, however, the use of these drugs in this fashion has failed to yield reliable and consistent results.

MEDICATION TO DECREASE PERFORMANCE

In racehorses, medication such as tranquilizers or depressants may be given in an effort to calm nervous or "washy" horses that may expend lots of energy in the paddock prior to a race. If the horses are calmer in the paddock, it is hoped that they will run better during the race. Also, such drugs might also be given to horses in an intentional effort to make them lose races; a long shot that wins a race can bring a handsome profit to the bettor who knew beforehand that the favorite was tranquilized. Of course, it's for exactly these reasons that the use of medication for such purposes is strictly prohibited by racing commissions.

In show horses, substances that induce tranquilization and cannot be detected are sought after by some people. In order to win competitions, show hunters not only have to jump fences, they have to jump in a calm and happy fashion (or at least the judges have to think that the horses are calm and happy). Unfortunately, calmness and happiness may not necessarily be the nature of a particular horse. And, some horses actually prefer staying in their stalls to jumping over a bunch of obstacles. Thus, medication may be given to a particular horse to help him overcome a completely rational "problem"—not liking to jump over fences in a calm and happy fashion.

Exercise, in the form of pre-competition longeing, for example, is one method of trying to make a horse tired, and therefore quieter, prior to his classes. However, many veterinarians and trainers fear that additional exercise, beyond what the horse gets in the competition, may ultimately increase wear and tear on the horse. They feel that this could conceivably lead to injury to the musculoskeletal system. (Longeing a horse prior to competition also means that the trainer has to be up really early.) Medication that provides mild sedation and tranquilization of the horse is an easy and seductive alternative. However, the use of tranquilizers—the obvious drug of choice for this "problem"—in this fashion is a violation of the rules of various horse show associations. Many other substances, which cannot be detected by routine drug tests are used to try to calm horses, but tryptophan, calcium, dexamethasone or ACTH have never shown any consistent calming effect, and are also clearly against the rules.

MEDICATION TO RESTORE PERFORMANCE
The use of medication to restore a horse's normal performance is certainly common. The rationale for use of medication in this fashion is easy to understand. For example, if a horse is experiencing some form of minor pain, he may limp and be reluctant or unable to perform in a normal fashion. An anti-inflammatory and pain-relieving agent would be expected to help restore the horse's normal performance by helping to alleviate the pain; if the horse doesn't hurt, he will be more likely to perform "normally."

A number of medications are used in this fashion. Nonsteroidal anti-inflammatory agents (NSAIDs), drugs such as phenylbutazone ("bute") that help relieve pain and inflammation, are among the drugs most commonly administered to horses. Similarly, if a horse's joint is sore and inflamed, injections of steroidal anti-inflammatory agents directly into the joint is a common way to help relieve inflammation and the resulting pain.

23

Medications such as these are clearly therapeutic. They are just as clearly overused. For example, not all horses that compete will become sore or lame as a result. However, many competition horses are often given anti-inflammatory drugs "just in case" they get sore. Or, they may receive "maintenance" injections in their joints, under the rather silly supposition that joints need some sort of pharmacological boost to perform at their best. There's certainly no medical reason to believe that such interventions are worthwhile for the horse. Furthermore, while medicating a horse in pain may be a rational thing to do from a therapeutic standpoint, medicating him just so that he can compete despite an injury may not be in the horse's best interest.

When horses compete, some people want to make sure that their horse has an "edge" on the competition. They also want to make sure that some other competitor doesn't have an "unfair" chemical advantage. Consequently, many competition horses end up floating in drugs that are supposed to "help" them perform in one way or another, if for no other reason than "because everyone else is doing it." What one person does, others seem to follow. In lemming-like fashion, it sometimes seems that if one successful trainer said that he was giving his horse a pint of motor oil every day, soon everyone in the area would be rushing to the auto parts store to stock up.

Even effective medication may have its downside. Local injections of steroidal anti-inflammatory agents into arthritic horse joints may allow the horse to continue to perform in the short term; however, continued indiscriminate use of steroids may be at the expense of the horse's future soundness (or life). Some unethical horse people will even anesthetize arthritic joints so that the horse does not feel a damaged joint at all. This practice is clearly dangerous to the horse and to the rider. It can result in total breakdown of the horse, who may be unable to feel, and therefore protect his leg. If the horse breaks down, the rider can also be seriously injured. Horse owners and trainers should consider the potential adverse consequences of unlimited or careless use of medication in horses.

Vitamin and mineral supplements are also commonly used to try to ensure that a horse is "normal" and in good health. While commonly used, no studies have shown that vitamin and mineral supplements are beneficial, or even necessary.

Endurance horses, for example, are frequently supplemented with *electrolytes*. Electrolytes are body salts that are lost in the horse's sweat. Supplementation with electrolytes certainly does not appear to be harmful for these horses; in fact, at least one study suggests that the administration of high concentrations of electrolytes, glucose and water may help delay fatigue. Providing adequate water, however, is the most important factor to consider for endurance horses and horses that compete in other high intensity sports.

In reality, getting optimum performance from your horse is not usually that complicated. The best thing that you can do for your horse to make sure that his performance is as good as is possible for him is to feed him well and provide good physical care.

"ACCIDENTAL" MEDICATION

Some of the medication given to horses can cause them to test positive for the presence of substances in the blood that are considered illegal by organizations that oversee competitions. For example, injections of procaine penicillin, a commonly used antibiotic, will cause horses to test positive for the presence of illegal anesthetic agents. Procaine is an anesthetic agent added to penicillin to take the sting out of its injection. Unfortunately, it is impossible for a drug test to tell the difference between injections of an antibiotic for therapeutic purposes and an illegally administered local anesthetic. (As discussed earlier, an anesthetic might be illegally given to make a sore area of the horse numb, so that he can compete without signs of lameness.) Similarly, guaifenesin, used as an expectorant in some cough preparations, can cause a falsely positive drug test for methocarbamol, a muscle relaxant.

Sometimes horses will "accidentally" test positive for drugs if they are given some otherwise benign substance. For example, cola drinks or chocolate can cause horses to test positive for caffeine, an illegal stimulant. Fortunately, this sort of thing doesn't happen very often.

Herbal products present another unique set of problems. Some plants have active pharmaceutical agents in them, and this can cause positive drug tests. Laboratory reports indicating positive tests for drugs such as ephedrine, phenylpropanolamine, pseudoephedrine, norpseudoephedrine and caffeine have been received by racing officials in horses that were given herbal or botanical products. For example, spinach octacosanol tablets were shown to be contaminated with phenylpropanolamine after a horse racing in California tested positive for phenylpropanolamine. Numerous trainers in the US have been penalized for positive tests for caffeine after administering various herbal products containing guarana to their horses. (Guarana, made from the crushed seed of a climbing shrub native to Brazil and Uruguay, is in fact used to prepare a hot beverage in those countries.) Some of these products are labeled "No added caffeine," although guarana is the obvious source of caffeine. Some ginseng-containing herbal products are known to contain sufficient caffeine to produce a positive test, as are products such as "Herbal Ecstasy." Various herbal products contain alkaloids from ephedra, a plant-based stimulant.

When drugs are given to a horse, the horse's system metabolizes them and removes them from his system. Depending on the drug, this can take from a period of days to months. Therefore, substances that are prohibited by organizations that oversee competitions should be used carefully. The horse owner and trainer must pay attention and make sure that the horse has had adequate time to let the drug clear his system. Of course, with plant-based products, where the constituents are mostly unknown, this can be a particular problem.

In horse shows overseen by the United States Equestrian Federation (USEF), a good way to ensure that drug detection does not become a problem is to "declare" that a drug has been given to a horse for therapeutic purposes prior to competition. The horse will be able to show twenty-four hours after the declared last time of administration of the drug. If he then tests positive for some substance, you will not be subject to penalties.

MEDICATION TO "MASK" DRUGS OR DILUTE OTHER MEDICATION

Some medication is given to horses in an effort to make it more difficult to detect other, prohibited drugs. In past years, substances such as thiamine (vitamin B$_1$) and dipyrone have been used as "masking" agents. Strangely, these drugs have never been shown to be effective in preventing detection of other drugs, so if you're inclined to use such things, it's certainly at your own risk.

Similarly, diuretics may be given to horses to avoid positive drug tests. Diuretics dilute the concentration of drugs in the urine by increasing the amount of water in it. However, this also is not a very effective way to get around drug tests. The effects of diuretics are quite rapid and transient, lasting only a few hours, and the use of diuretics is generally controlled or prohibited by the various organizations.

THE REGULATION OF MEDICATION IN PERFORMANCE HORSES

Performance horses are subjected to a mind-numbing array of regulations, depending on the organization that oversees the competitions. It would be virtually impossible to detail all of the individual rules and regulations regarding the use of drugs and medication for each horse organization. Each organization has its own rules, and those rules are subject to constant modification. In the case of racehorses, the medication rules vary in each state (there are now 43 states that have pari-mutuel racing).

Drug rules reflect the different philosophies of the various organizations. Bodies such as the Jockey Club, the Fédération Equestre Internationale (FEI) and the American Quarter Horse Association (AQHA) tend to be the most strict. Their view is that horses should not be in an event if they have detectable levels of any drug in their systems. At the other end of the spectrum, the National Cutting Horse Association (NCHA) and the National Reining Horse Association (NRHA) of the United States don't have any rules prohibiting the use of foreign substances in horses (although the NCHA does not allow the administration of any drugs to horses in the ring, except in emergency situations).

The use of most drugs in racehorses is prohibited. Most states have specific regulations that allow the use of phenylbutazone (and other nonsteroidal anti-inflammatory drugs) and furosemide. The states often differ, however, in how they approach the problem of medication control. In New York State, certain drugs may or may not be given within a certain period of time prior to post. For example, antihistamines must not be given within 48 hours of post time. In the state of California, the regulations are written specifically defining the permitted amounts or levels of drugs in the horse. These rules are similar to rules regarding blood alcohol levels in people; it doesn't really matter how much you had to drink or when you drank it—if your blood alcohol level is above the legal limit, you're sunk. It is literally impossible to know whether a particular horse's level of a certain drug will be within acceptable levels after a specific period of time without actually testing him. When a drug is given to a horse, it is removed from the system at a relatively constant rate; this rate varies with the individual horse. Blood or urine levels of drugs such as phenylbutazone above those permitted may subject the owner and trainer to sanctions from the racing commission. Kentucky has yet another approach to the control of medication: horses cannot run on tranquilizers, stimulants, depressants, local anesthetics or narcotics. All other drugs are considered therapeutic, and their use is permitted under veterinary supervision.

The drug rules of the United States Equestrian Federation, the largest regulatory body overseeing show horses in the United States, are the most complex of all of the organizations. The USEF tests thousands of horses every year (and spends millions of dollars a year doing so) in an effort to ensure that horse show competitions are fair. The rules of the USEF are subject to constant review and change. It is important that competitors, trainers and veterinarians involved with show horses be aware of the changing and sometimes convoluted nature of the drug rules.

Most horses competing under USEF rules are subject to its "Therapeutic Substance" provisions, with the exception of endurance horses, which compete under "No Foreign Substance" provisions. The USEF categorizes drugs into two groups. The first group of com-pounds are *forbidden* substances. These are substances that might affect the performance of horses and/or ponies. This group includes literally thousands of substances, including stimulants, tranquilizers, local anesthetics and depressants (see Table 1, p. 29).

If a horse or pony has been given a forbidden substance, but it has been used for a *therapeutic* purpose such as treating or diagnosing an illness or injury, the use of the substance has to be "declared" at the show (the show secretary should know what needs to be done), and the horse must be withheld from competition for twenty-four hours. If the horse or pony has been given a forbidden substance for a *non-therapeutic* purpose, such as for trailering or clipping, then the horse must be withheld from showing until no trace of the drug

TABLE 1

A Few Examples of the Many Substances that are Forbidden by the United States Equestrian Federation (USEF) Drugs and Medications Rule

Acepromazine	Dantrolene	Nitroglycerin
Albuterol	Diazepam	Opiates
Aminophylline	Ephedrine	Pentoxyfylline
Antihistamines	Epinephrine	Phenobarbitol
Apomorphine	Fluphenazine	Phenylpropanolamine
Barbituates	Furosemide	Procaine Penicillin
Benzocaine	Guaifenesin	Reserpine
Beta Blockers	Hydroxyzine	Scopolamine
Bupivicaine	Ketamine	Tramadol
Caffeine	Lidocaine	Valerian
Carprofen	Lithium	Xylazine
Codeine	Morphine	Xylocaine

United States Equestrian Federation, "Drugs and Medications Guidelines," April 1, 2006. http://www.usef.org/documents/drugsMeds/USEF_EquineDrugsMedicationsPamphlet.pdf (accessed March 1, 2007).

remains in the animal's system; this can take a few days, depending on the drug.

The second group of drugs are those substances that have quantitative restrictions. These are drugs that can be in the horse at the time that he is showing, but only in certain amounts. That is, the USEF restricts the amounts of these drugs that can be given to the horse. This group of drugs includes (but is not limited to) such substances as phenylbutazone and flunixin meglumine (two of the most commonly used nonsteroidal anti-inflammatory drugs), methocarbamol, and many corticosteroid anti-inflammatory agents. The USEF provides guidelines to competitors for the use of these drugs. For example, phenylbutazone and flunixin cannot be used at the same time, and the USEF recommends that, if one of these compounds is used, you wait seven days before using the other if you are planning on going to a USEF show during that time. The USEF also gives recommended doses and withdrawal times for substances with quantitative restrictions.

Insofar as herbal or other "natural" products go, the USEF explicitly warns that these products may contain or be contaminated by substances that could cause a horse or pony to test positive for a forbidden substance in USEF sanctioned competitions, and recommends that owners and trainers be skeptical about claims that a particular preparation is "legal," "permissable" or "untestable." Products such as valerian, kava kava, chamomile and devil's claw are just a few of the botanical preparations that can cause horses to test positive. The USEF also advises that it does not endorse any such products (and asks that if you see a "natural" product that claims to be USEF sanctioned, you call the USEF and tell them about it).

It is very important that the individual competitor or trainer be familiar with the rules that apply to his or her particular sport in order to avoid disqualification or suspension from competition. Due to the sometimes vague and ever-changing nature of drug regulations, close consultation with your trainer, veterinarian and/or overseeing competition body is strongly recommended. The best way to avoid problems regarding allowable levels of drugs in your performance horse is to know the rules.

CHAPTER

Medications, Herbs and Supplements for the Horse

—— A ——

ABSORBINE® (see Liniment)

ACEPROMAZINE MALEATE ("Ace")

Acepromazine maleate (ace-PRO-ma-zine MAL-ee-ate) is a commonly prescribed tranquilizer. Its effects are generally milder than other tranquilizers used in horses but may be somewhat longer lasting. There are reports of tranquilization lasting up to twenty-four hours in some horses (although most horses seem tranquilized for only a few hours).

Acepromazine is available in a sterile solution, which may be given by intramuscular (IM) or intravenous (IV) injection. The sterile solution can also be squirted into the mouth where it is absorbed through the mucous membranes of the gums. Acepromazine maleate is also available in oral tablets. A related product, promazine granules, is given in the feed (see Promazine Hydrochloride, p. 160).

Precautions
Tranquilization of horses with acepromazine may lead to a false sense of security when working around them. Horses that are tranquilized can still react quickly to external stimuli. Horses maintain their visual and hearing capacities while on acepromazine, so loud sounds or rapid movements should be avoided. The drug has little, if any, pain-relieving effect. Painful procedures should be avoided while using this drug.

Acepromazine is not a very potent tranquilizer. If a horse really objects to something, such as body clipping or trailering, acepromazine may not provide enough tranquilization to get the job done, no matter how much is used. To increase the tranquilizing effect, sometimes acepromazine is used in combination with other tranquilizers, such as xylazine or detomodine (see Xylazine, p. 198, and Detomodine, p. 78).

Horses intended for use in shows must not have traces of this drug in their systems.

Side Effects

In addition to its tranquilizing effects, acepromazine is a potent dilator of the small peripheral blood vessels of the horse's body. Because of this side effect, it is occasionally prescribed for the treatment of laminitis in an effort to improve or increase circulation to the feet. This effect on blood vessels is also responsible for decreased blood pressure and sudden fainting in some horses that have been given the drug.

Acepromazine causes relaxation of the muscles of the penis in male horses. An unfortunate side effect, partial paralysis of the muscles of the penis, has been described. Horses so affected may be unable to retract their penis. Although this complication is extremely rare, this side effect may be a consideration if the drug is to be used in breeding stallions.

ACTH (Adrenocorticotropic Hormone)

ACTH is a hormone that serves as a stimulator of the *adrenal glands*. The adrenal glands lie next to the kidneys, hence, the name *ad* ("next to") *renal* ("kidney"). The adrenal glands produce a number of hormones important for normal metabolic functions in the horse. ACTH is available as a sterile gel, which is given by intramuscular (IM) administration.

ACTH is manufactured as a diagnostic aid to help determine if there is a problem with adrenal gland function in dogs and cats. However, the drug is used in horses in an effort to stimulate the release of *cortisol* into the horse's body. Some people feel that higher levels of plasma cortisol ("natural" steroids) may make a horse feel calmer. There is no medical evidence to support this use of the drug and no studies have been done to document its effects.

Indiscriminate use of ACTH in horses is not advisable. There is a potential to deplete or adversely affect the adrenal gland through its use in this fashion. Prolonged use of ACTH, causing elevated levels of cortisol in the body, can potentially cause the same effects as Equine Cushing's Disease (ECD).

ACETAZOLAMIDE
Acetazolamide (a-cee-ta-ZO-la-mide) is a diuretic agent that is used for the treatment of *hyperkalemic periodic paralysis (HYPP)*. HYPP, a condition that occurs in horses carrying bloodlines that trace back to the Quarter Horse sire Impressive, is caused by an abnormality in the horse's body that causes it to be unable to control its electrolytes in a normal fashion (see Electrolytes, p. 90). Acetazolamide increases potassium excretion from the kidney, and thereby helps normalize electrolyte levels, and also affects glucose metabolism.

Proper dietary management is essential for management of horses with HYPP, with or without drug therapy.

ADEQUAN® (see Polysulfated Glycosaminoglycan)

ADRENALINE (see Epinephrine)

ALCOHOL
The term alcohol refers to the chemical configuration of a number of substances. There are literally dozens of alcohols. The two main alcohols that find use in the equine world are *isopropyl alcohol* and *ethyl alcohol* (see Isopropyl Alcohol, p. 119, and Ethyl Alcohol, p. 95).

Alcohols are used primarily as solvents to dissolve other substances. As such, they have a variety of pharmacological uses. Isopropyl alcohol ("rubbing alcohol") can be used to remove things from the skin, such as tape residue or some oily substances. In people, it can be used to bathe the skin for the purpose of cooling; it does this by evaporating quickly, causing a cooling effect. In high concentrations alcohol is an irritant to the skin.

In horses, both isopropyl and ethyl alcohol are used to formulate a number of preparations such as liniments, wound treatments and hoof dressings (see Liniment, p. 126, Wound Treatments, p. 196, and Hoof Dressings, p. 111). Some people apply alcohol directly to the horse's legs after exercise, presumably as some sort of liniment or coolant. The actual effects of such treatment are unknown.

Alcohol baths are recommended by some veterinarians in an attempt to reduce fever in sick horses. Due to its rapid evaporation and subsequent cooling effect, alcohol may work well in this regard.

Alcohol is a good *antiseptic* (local anti-infective) for the skin, killing bacteria by dehydrating them as it dries. However, swabbing the skin with alcohol prior to local injection does little apparent good unless the area is allowed to dry first; otherwise, the local skin bacteria in the swabbed area are merely suspended in a solution of alcohol. Thus, it may theoretically be easier to contaminate the underlying tissue if the skin over the area is swabbed with alcohol first. That is, it may be easier to get bacteria under the skin if they're in a solution as opposed to lying directly on the surface of the skin. In practice, it probably doesn't really matter if you swab an injection site with alcohol or not.

Ethyl alcohol is sometimes used to "block" peripheral nerves, particularly to the feet and tail of horses. The alcohol removes the myelin covering from the nerves, which makes the nerves function poorly. The use of ethyl alcohol for such purposes is generally considered unethical by breed organizations, and some, such as the American Quarter Horse Association (AQHA), test to see if horses have blocked tails.

Ethyl alcohol is also being investigated for possible use desensitizing arthritic joints. If proven safe and effective, it would not promote a cure, but it would possibly help relieve suffering in painful joints for which there is no other therapeutic option.

ALLANTOIN

In people, allantoin (a-LAN-toe-in) is used in an effort to promote healing and tissue repair. It is used in the treatment of various skin conditions, such as wounds and skin infections. In World War I, it was noticed that wounds that were infested with maggots healed better than those that had no maggot infestation; the maggots were discovered to produce allantoin. Once the active agent was identified, it became possible to use allantoin (instead of maggots) to promote healing.

Allantoin is available as an ingredient in an over-the-counter hoof dressing (see Hoof Dressings, p. 111).

ALMOND OIL

Almond oil is obtained by pressing almonds. It has some use as an emollient (see Emollient, p. 90) and is contained in some hoof dressings (see Hoof Dressings, p. 111).

ALOE (Aloe Vera)

There are over 200 varieties of plants that produce aloe, a sticky juice obtained from the leaves. Aloe vera is a common house plant. The juice from this plant is commonly applied to cuts and burns, where it is reported to have emollient effects (see Emollient, p. 90). It is also reported to speed healing. Plant aloes are also used as *cathartics* (stimulants to the intestines that cause evacuation of the bowels) in people.

The relevant parts of aloe plants are the *gel* and *latex*. Aloe gel is the clear, jelly-like substance obtained from the slimy cells in the center of the leaf. Aloe latex is obtained from the cells just beneath the leaf skin.

In the 1960s in Japan, a study was done that suggested that aloe could speed healing of damaged skin. More recently, study groups from the US Food and Drug Administration (USFDA) have looked at the tests done on aloe and concluded that there is no good evidence for this. One study of an aloe-containing dressing applied to surgical wounds in people found that the dressing actually delayed healing.

Aloe vera is commonly applied to wounds of the horse and is available in a number of over-the-counter preparations for this purpose (see Wound Treatments, p. 196). It is also found in some hoof dressing products (see Hoof Dressings, p. 111).

ALTRENOGEST (Regu-Mate®)

Altrenogest is a *progestin*. Progestins are used to prevent *estrus* ("heat") in mares and in the management of breeding mares.

Altrenogest is commonly used in show mares to keep them from coming into heat (with all its reported behavioral side effects, real or imagined) during competition. In the management of broodmares, altrenogest is commonly given in an effort to help them maintain pregnancy. However, there is no indication that mares fail to maintain pregnancy due to deficiencies in progesterone.

Altrenogest has been used in attempts to synchronize breeding cycles (that is, to try to get mares to come into heat at particular times). Altrenogest is also used to help regulate transitional mares. Mares have a breeding season; that is, there is a time that they can be bred and a time when they do not come into heat. Frequently, when their heat cycle begins and ends, it is irregular, with unpredictable patterns of prolonged heat. Altrenogest has been used to modulate this activity and to encourage the beginning of a more normal heat cycle (see Progesterone, p. 159).

Some people have advocated the use of altrenogest to try to alter the mood of unruly male horses, too. There is no clinical data to support this use of the drug, although it seems to have little chance of being harmful to geldings. Long-term use of altrenogest in stallions may depress their fertility.

Precautions
Altrenogest can be absorbed through human skin and has the potential to affect the menstrual cycle of women administering the drug. Latex gloves should be worn to protect the hands and prevent skin absorption. Pregnant women should not handle altrenogest.

Side Effects
Altrenogest is remarkably safe and associated with no significant side effects. Neither altrenogest nor any other progestin should be used in mares that have previously had or are currently exhibiting signs of uterine infection or inflammation because it may make the problem worse.

ALUM
Alum has been around since the days of the ancient Greeks. Alum is a powerful astringent and has mild antiseptic properties (see Astringent, p. 45, and Antiseptic, p. 43). Human athletes use it to toughen their skin. It is also used to stop blood flow. Alum is a principal component of styptic pencils, used to stop bleeding after people cut themselves shaving.

In horses, alum is found in some wound dressings, where it is presumably used to help stop or prevent surface bleeding (see Wound Treatments, p. 196).

ALUMINUM SULFATE
Aluminum sulfate is a powerful astringent, much like alum (see Alum, p. 36, and Astringent, p. 45). It is widely used to make antiperspirant products for people.

Aluminum sulfate is a component of a coolant gel available for use on horse legs (see Coolant Gel, p. 69). Presumably, its astringent effects may make the skin of the leg seem "tighter." It is unlikely to have any other effects on the horse's leg.

AMIKACIN SULFATE (Amiglyde-V®)
Amikacin is one of a group of antibiotics known as the *aminoglycosides*. These antibiotics kill bacteria by interfering with mechanisms involved in bacterial reproduction.

Amikacin comes as a sterile solution that can be administered by intramuscular (IM) or intravenous (IV) injection. It is commonly used to treat intrauterine infection in mares. It is also added to substances injected into joints in an effort to reduce the risk of infection from such procedures. Amikacin is resistant to most of the enzymes that bacteria produce that inactivate other drugs of the same class.

Precautions
Amikacin is an effective drug when used as directed; however, its use is often limited by its cost.

Side Effects
Aminoglycoside antibiotics (like amikacin) have two primary side effects. First, they can damage the centers of hearing and balance in the brain. Second, they may impair function of the kidneys. Although these side effects are rare, horses that may have reduced kidney function (such as those that are dehydrated) or that are very young with immature kidneys should be monitored closely if this drug is chosen to treat an infection. Care should be taken when amikacin is used with nonsteroidal anti-inflammatory drugs (NSAIDs) because of the increased potential for kidney-related side effects.

AMINO ACID
Amino acids are the "letters of the alphabet" from which protein "words" are made (proteins are the structural components that

make up most of the body's tissue) as well as major components of body enzymes and many hormones. Twenty amino acids have been identified for normal growth and tissue formation, although more than twenty exist. Some of these are "essential"; that is, the horse must get them in some form in his diet. The requirements for specific amino acids have not been determined; however, the "normal" horse diet appears to supply adequate amounts of all amino acids required.

There is certainly no evidence that would suggest that specific amino acid supplementation is important in horses. Nor have amino acid deficiencies ever been identified as a problem in the horse. While a variety of products containing amino acids are available to give to horses, many of which claim a whole host of beneficial properties, in practice amino acids have little, if any, therapeutic value. Just because a horse needs some amino acids doesn't mean that more of them is necessarily better. Excess protein and amino acids are digested by the horse and used for energy; they are an expensive source of energy. And in fact, some studies in other animal species have shown that taking unusually large amounts of amino acids can create amino acid imbalances in the animal's body.

AMINOCAPROIC ACID (Amicar®)

Aminocaproic acid helps prevent blood clot breakdown in the human body. It is used in human medicine to help treat bleeding, especially when the bleeding occurs after dental surgery (particularly in patients that have blood clotting disorders). It is also sometimes given before an operation to prevent serious bleeding in patients with medical problems that increase the chance of bleeding.

Because of its effects in other species, it's been used in an effort to prevent bleeding from the lungs in heavily exercising horses (*exercise-induced pulmonary hemorrhage* or *"bleeders"*). There is no scientific proof of the efficacy or safety of aminocaproic acid and there would seem to be little justification for its race-day use.

AMINOPHYLLINE

In people, aminophylline (am-ih-NOFF-uh-lin) is sometimes used to treat the wheezing and shortness of breath that accompany such conditions as emphysema or asthma.

Unfortunately, in horses, aminophylline has a fairly narrow window of effective dosing range—that is, the dose at which the drug is not effective is not very different from the dose where unwanted side effects are seen. Thus, the drug is not widely used in horses.

AMMONIUM CHLORIDE
Ammonium chloride is a salt. It has some pharmaceutical use as an expectorant (see Expectorant, p. 96) and is found in some cough preparations for horses.

AMPICILLIN SODIUM (Amp-Equine®)
Ampicillin is an antibiotic used for the treatment of a variety of infections in the horse. It is one of a group of broad-spectrum penicillins, antibiotics that are chemically related to penicillin but that have the ability to kill more kinds of bacteria than does penicillin alone. The drugs work by disrupting the cell wall that surrounds certain bacteria, which destroys them.

Ampicillin comes as a dehydrated, sterile powder and is mixed, usually with sterile water, prior to intravenous (IV) or intramuscular (IM) injection. The drug can also be infused into the uterus of the mare to treat infection there. Oral forms of ampicillin can be used in some species, but the drug is not well-absorbed orally in the horse.

Side Effects
Ampicillin has few adverse properties. It should not be used in horses that are allergic to penicillin.

ANABOLIC STEROID
The word *anabolic* refers to building up or constructive processes of cells and tissues. Anabolic steroids are drugs that relate to the sex hormones. Anabolic effects of a drug include improvement of appetite, increased vigor, improvement in musculature and improvement in the hair coat. These drugs may be useful in conditions where there has been marked muscle tissue breakdown or general debilitation, such as with disease, prolonged anorexia or overwork.

Anabolic steroids are also associated with the typical expressions of aggressive, stallion-like behavior in horses. In addition, interference with normal estrous cycles is seen in mares maintained on anabolic steroids. Finally, a recent report associates long-term administration of anabolic steroids with dysfunction of the adrenal gland in one horse.

Some people use anabolic steroids to try to enhance performance in horses by building muscle or increasing aggressiveness. While the potential to improve performance with these drugs may be there, one study in Scotland failed to show any actual improvement in racehorses treated with these drugs.

Anabolic steroids are closely controlled by the US Food and Drug Administration (USFDA) because of their potential for abuse by humans.

ANTHELCIDE-EQ® (see Benzimidazole)

ANTIBACTERIAL
A substance that destroys bacteria or suppresses their reproduction or growth is an antibacterial.

Antibiotics (see below) have antibacterial effects. Antibacterial compounds used in the treatment of infectious conditions of the horse, such as sulfa drugs, are chemicals that are synthesized in the laboratory (see Sulfa, p. 178). Antibiotics come from naturally occurring microorganisms.

ANTIBIOTIC
An antibiotic is a chemical substance that is produced by a microorganism. This substance has the capacity, when provided in dilute solutions, to inhibit the growth of (*bacteriostatic*) or to kill (*bactericodal*) other microorganisms. Antibiotics that are sufficiently nontoxic to the host are used in the treatment of many diseases of the horse.

ANTIHISTAMINE
Antihistamines are drugs that work to block the effects of *histamine*, a naturally occurring chemical in the horse's body. It seems to have very important effects in the transmission of nerve impulses and in the control of secretions in the stomach.

Histamine is also one of many chemicals that are released during the process of inflammation. It has potent effects on the circulatory system of the horse. In addition to participating in the process of inflammation, histamine is involved in allergic shock (*anaphylaxis*), allergies and some types of adverse reactions to drugs. Histamine release is associated with swelling of tissue (such as is seen with *hives*) and itching, among other effects. When skin is scratched, the characteristic resulting redness is due to histamine.

Certain cells have specific locations on them that cause them to respond to histamine. Antihistamines block the effects of histamine by occupying these locations on the cells. Antihistamines do not remove the histamine from the cell sites, they only help to prevent further histamine binding to the cell sites.

Antihistamines are useful in countering the effects of histamine in many locations. In horses, they are most commonly used in the treatment of allergic reactions; they help counteract the swelling and itching that are commonly associated with these conditions. Preparations containing antihistamines are sometimes used for treatment of allergic respiratory conditions in horses and coughing. Some veterinarians have used antihistamine preparations for the treatment of laminitis. The pharmacological basis for this is not clear. Direct infusion of histamine into the horse does not cause laminitis.

Cimetidine, ranitidine and omeprazole are specific types of histamine blocking agents used for the treatment and control of gastric ulceration in horses and foals. Cimetidine has also been reported to be occasionally effective for treatment of a certain type of equine melanoma, a generally benign skin cancer (see Cimetidine, p. 66, Ranitidine, p. 166, and Omeprazole, p. 142).

Antihistamine preparations are available in sterile solution for intramuscular (IM) administration or in pill form for oral administration in the horse (see Hydroxyzine, p. 116, Pyrilamine, p. 165, and Tripelennamine, p. 186). These drugs are relatively nontoxic at recommended doses.

Comment
Antihistamine agents by themselves are frequently ineffective in treating or controlling allergies because many other agents besides histamine are involved in allergic reactions. Antihistamines only help control the symptoms of histamine-associated disease. Therefore, to get a cure, therapy must also be aimed at removing the cause of the problem.

ANTIOXIDANT

A popular nutrition buzzword is "antioxidant." Every supplement so labeled is seen as having only an upside and no downside. This is a myth. The claim is that these compounds seek out and remove *free radicals*, reactive chemicals that are produced during the process of inflammation and that are not even necessarily a bad thing. For example, free radicals play an important role in a number of biological processes, some of which are necessary for life, such as the intracellular killing of bacteria by white blood cells. Still, in excessive amounts, free radicals can cause harm to tissue, and the horse's body has a number of mechanisms to minimize free-radical-induced damage, and to repair damage that does occur.

Ensuring your horse's health is not simply a matter of giving him more antioxidants. In fact, antioxidant compounds such as vitamins A, C and E are not necessarily benign, nor are they "pure" antioxidants (see Vitamin A, p. 189, Vitamin C, p. 193, and Vitamin E, p. 193). Rather, such compounds are what are known as *redox* (oxidation-reduction) agents.

In chemical terms, redox reactions primarily involve the transfer of electrons between two chemical species. In fact, redox reactions can go both ways. That is, in some circumstances, compounds may tend to be *antioxidant* (for example, in the physiologic quantities found in food); however, such substances can also be *pro-oxidant*, producing billions of harmful free radicals, particularly when provided in the quantities found in some supplements. For example, in humans, excess vitamin C from supplements mobilizes harmless ferric iron stored in the body and converts it to harmful ferrous iron, which induces damage to the heart and other organs. (Supplemental vitamin E and C have not been shown to be of benefit in preventing heart disease in people.)

The biggest problem of all is that nobody knows what the defining characteristics are that make a given chemical an "antioxidant." So, when people talk about antioxidants, and their wonderful effects, and why you need to feed them to your horse, take into consideration that they're out on a limb that may not be attached to a tree.

ANTISEPTIC

An antiseptic is a product that is used to kill or stop the growth of bacteria. The term is always used to refer to products that are used on living tissue. Most antiseptic agents are used to clean the skin of the horse.

ARNICA

Arnica is an herb derived from one of a variety of plants of the genus *Arnica*. In herbal medicine, a tincture of the dried flowers is sometimes applied externally in an effort to help reduce pain and inflammation resulting from bruises and sprains.

Arnica is included as a component of a coolant gel sold over-the-counter for application to horse limbs (see Coolant Gel, p. 69). There is no indication that the preparation is effective in horses.

ARQUEL® (see Meclofenamic Acid)

ASPIRIN

Aspirin was first introduced in 1899. It is one of the oldest pain relievers and anti-inflammatory drugs used in medicine. Its effects are, in general, quite mild. It can be used as a reliever of mild to moderate pain, primarily of muscular or skeletal pain (such as arthritis), and as an agent to control or reduce fever.

Aspirin also tends to inhibit the aggregation (collecting together) of *platelets*, the cells in the blood that start the first stages of blood clotting. That's why people say that aspirin "thins the blood." Because of this effect on the blood platelets, the use of aspirin is advocated by some veterinarians as an aid in the treatment of laminitis in an effort to help prevent the formation of blood clots in the circulatory system of the hoof. Aspirin is also advocated by some veterinary ophthalmologists as a good choice for relief of inflammation of the eye.

Aspirin tablets, boluses or powder are available for oral administration in the horse. It is fairly inexpensive.

Precautions

Horses with known liver or kidney damage should be monitored closely if on aspirin. Aspirin should not be used in conjunction with aminoglycoside antibiotics (e.g., gentamycin sulfate or amikacin sulfate) because it increases the potential for these drugs to have toxic effects on the kidneys (see Gentamycin Sulfate, p. 105, and Amikacin Sulfate, p. 37). Caution should be used in giving aspirin to weak, anemic, dehydrated or debilitated animals. It is also recommended that aspirin not be given to animals for two weeks prior to surgery so that blood clotting is not affected. Animals under 30 days of age have difficulty in metabolizing and eliminating aspirin.

Side Effects
Aspirin has the potential to cause gastrointestinal ulceration, particularly in large doses. The drug should not be used in horses with ulcers.

Comment
In spite of its long history, aspirin has not found widespread use in horses as a pain reliever. Other nonsteroidal anti-inflammatory drugs seem to be much more effective in horses for the relief of pain and inflammation (see Nonsteroidal Anti-Inflammatory Drug, p. 141).

ASTRAGALUS
The flowering plant genus *Astragalus* (a-STRAG-a-lus) makes up the largest genus of vascular plants—plants that have specialized tissues for conducting water—on Earth. Better known by such common names as "milkvetch" or "locoweed," the genus contains 2,500 mostly perennial species distributed primarily around the northern hemisphere and South America.

Various *Astragalus* species may be included in herbal products intended to "boost" a horse's immune system. While the product appears to be safe, there's no evidence that it's effective for any of its therapeutic purposes (which, in humans, include such conditions as the common cold and upper respiratory infections).

Comment
The recorded history of *Astragalus* dates back at least to the first century A.D., and the genus was well known to western European botanists of the seventeenth century. A number of species of *Astragalus* have properties valuable in ice creams, lotions and pharmaceuticals. A few species are edible or have medicinal uses, and some are used for livestock forage. However, a large number of North American species are poisonous, especially to livestock and

wildlife, a property due to the accumulation of selenium from soils or synthesis of high levels of certain toxins and alkaloids in the foliage. The toxicity is characterized by bizarre behavior, hence the name "locoweed" (*loco* is Spanish for "crazy") given to many species.

ASTRINGENT

Astringent means "causing contraction." Astringent agents are generally applied to the skin. An astringent agent dries and tightens the skin.

In horses, astringents are applied to the skin surface. The effects of an astringent are limited to the skin and they have no effect on the underlying tissues. Astringents work by causing the surface proteins, which are normally in solution, to settle down into solid particles (this process is called *precipitation*). This can cause the tissue to contract, wrinkle and harden. In high concentrations, astringent substances can be very irritating to the skin.

Therapeutically, astringents can be used to stop bleeding and reduce inflamed mucous membranes. They may have some effect in promoting wound healing, presumably through antiseptic effects (see Antiseptic, p. 43).

ATROPINE

Atropine is a drug that, when given systemically, has a variety of effects on the nervous system of the horse. Although it may be more frequently used in other species, atropine is rarely used systemically in the horse due to its side effects. However, atropine ointment is commonly used in treatment of eye inflammation in horses. Atropine causes the eye muscles to relax and dilate, which helps relieve the pain and spasm associated with eye inflammation.

Atropine injections have been used by some veterinarians for treatment of toxicities from organophosphate compounds. It is also an old treatment for colic, since atropine stops intestinal cramping by stopping intestinal movement. But, when atropine is used for treatment of these conditions in horses, it may shut down the movement of the intestines with potentially fatal consequences. In fact, atropine injections to healthy horses (those not experiencing a colic episode) can cause the intestines to completely shut down, too.

45

AZITHROMYCIN

Azithromycin (a-zith-ro-MY-sin) is an antibiotic that finds its most common use in the treatment of bacterial pneumonia caused by *Rhodococcus equi* in foals. Azithromycin is a subclass of the medication called *macrolide antibiotics*. It was only discovered in 1980, and it is derived from erythromycin, although it differs from that drug chemically (see Erythromycin, p. 94). It works by stopping the growth of bacteria by interfering with the bacteria's ability to make proteins. When compared to erythromycin, the drug lasts longer in the horse's system and so can be administered less frequently.

Azithromycin is commonly administered with rifampin for the treatment of R. equi infection (see Rifampin, p. 167).

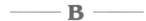

B

BACITRACIN (Neosporin®, Triple Antibiotic Ointment®, Neobacimyx®)

Bacitracin is an antibiotic that blocks specific reactions that are needed for certain bacteria to make their cell walls. Bacitracin is available in ointment formulations for applications to wound surfaces or to the surface of the eye. It cannot be given orally, because it is not absorbed from the GI tract, and it cannot be given systemically because it is toxic.

Bacitracin is almost always combined with two other antibiotics, neomycin and polymixin B (see Neomycin, p. 138, and Polymixin B, p. 154). This combination increases the numbers of bacteria killed when compared to those killed by each antibiotic individually. Some studies have shown that the rate of wound healing is increased in wounds treated with this combination of antibiotics. Bacitracin, along with other antibiotics, is also frequently mixed with corticosteroid anti-inflammatory agents (see Corticosteroid, p. 71).

BACTERIAL SUPPLEMENTS

A number of different bacteria are normally found in the intestinal tract in horses. Some species of intestinal bacteria (such as *E. coli*), while normally present in the intestine, have also been associated with disease states. Other types of intestinal bacteria have not yet been associated with disease and are therefore presumed to be beneficial. In people, for example, *Lactobacillus* species have gained favor in the "natural" health market as being of benefit in the digestive process, in particular in aiding in the digestion of protein.

A variety of nutritional supplements are available for the horse that contain one or more types of dried or live bacteria, including *Lactobacillus, Streptococcus* and *Bacillus* species. These bacteria are supposed to help the horse digest his feed more efficiently and help provide his intestines with a constant supply of "beneficial" bacteria.

There is absolutely no evidence that feeding bacterial supplements to horses is of any benefit. In fact, there are more questions about bacterial supplements than there are answers. For example, good research has determined that living bacteria can't exist in a supplement container or tube for long. For bacteria to grow, reproduce and survive, they require a relatively constant supply of fresh nutrients that could not be provided in a small container. It's hard to imagine how feeding a horse dead bacteria could be of benefit to the horse. If the bacteria are dried, as in some products, are they then still active? How can or do the bacteria survive the perilous journey through the horse's stomach, where the environment is so acidic that relatively few bacteria are able to live there under normal circumstances? Because of such questions, supplementation with bacteria is rarely taken seriously by equine nutritionists. Fortunately, bacterial supplements do not seem to cause the horse any harm.

Most frequently, several bacterial species are combined in supplements. One human "natural healing" source suggests that supplementation with a variety of different bacteria is not advisable. It says that the various bacteria may antagonize each other.

In reality, since it is unlikely that bacterial supplementation is of any benefit or harm, it may all just be a moot, though expensive, point.

BALSAM (Balsam of Fir, Balsam of Peru)

A balsam is a *resin*. Resins are solid or semisolid substances that ooze forth from plants or from insects feeding on plants.

The active ingredients in most balsams are two acids, *benzoic* and *cinnamic*. Balsams can be used as local skin irritants and are used in the preparation of some wound dressings in the hope that they will stimulate the growth of surface epithelial cells of the skin (see

47

Wound Treatment, p. 196). In people, balsams are occasionally used for the treatment of bedsores.

BANAMINE® (see Flunixin Meglumine)

BAYTRIL® (see Enrofloxacin)

BECLOMETHASONE DIPROPIONATE (Beconase®)

Beclomethasone dipropionate (beck-lo-METH-a-zone di-PRO-pea-o-nate) is an inhaled corticosteroid drug (see Corticosteroid, p. 71), used with inhalers designed for horses in the treatment of airway problems such as *chronic obstructive pulmonary disease (COPD)*. Inhaled steroids are a very effective treatment for inflamed air passages; the inhaled route of administration is considered a *topical* application of the drugs.

Because beclomethasone is applied topically to the airway passages, the dose of steroids is quite low, compared to what is necessary when steroids are given by other routes of administration for the treatment of airway disease. A lower dose is typically associated with fewer side effects in the administration of any drug.

BEE POLLEN

Bee pollen is a fine, powderlike material that is produced by flowering plants. Bees gather it to make honey.

Bee pollen contains vitamins B and C, some trace minerals and protein. While these things are needed in the horse diet, routine feeding should supply ample amounts of them for the horse.

In people, bee pollen has been promoted to increase energy levels. Studies in people have shown no benefit of bee pollen on athletic performance. In fact, some people may be allergic it.

Dramatic claims of healthful benefits from bee pollen for the horse cannot be substantiated.

BENTONITE

Bentonite is a natural earthen clay. It is used in the manufacture of various hoof preparations (see Hoof Dressings, p. 111). It has no proven therapeutic value.

BENZALKONIUM CHLORIDE (Fungisan®)

Benzalkonium chloride is an all-purpose antibacterial agent and a mild astringent (see Antibacterial, p. 40, and Astringent, p. 45). It is the principal ingredient in a commonly used over-the-counter skin preparation for treatment of skin infections of the horse.

Benzalkonium chloride has no effect against viruses or bacterial spores. Importantly, it is inactivated by soaps, which (unfortunately) are commonly applied to wash the surface of the horse's skin prior to application of this product.

When applied to the skin, benzalkonium chloride tends to form a film over the bacteria living on the surface. The bacteria can remain alive under this film. Tissue debris also inactivates benzalkonium chloride, so it has limited effectiveness in areas where tissue fluids are being secreted or on wounds.

BENZIMIDAZOLE

Many varieties of benzimidazole (ben-zi-ma-DAY-zol) dewormers are available for the control of internal parasites in the horse. Pharmacologists have investigated literally hundreds of variations of this type of product. Preparations are available for the horse for administration in the feed, by oral paste or in a liquid for *nasogastric intubation* (stomach tube).

Benzimidazole drugs that are commonly used in the horse include thiabendazole, oxfendazole, mebendazole, oxibendazole and fenbendazole. All of these drugs act in the same fashion, by interfering with the energy-generating mechanisms of the parasites. The drug kills parasites over a two- to three-day period.

In increased doses, benzimidazoles also kill parasite larvae (as does ivermectin, another deworming agent, see p. 120). Killing the immature larvae before they reach the adult stage in the intestines is of obvious benefit. Thiabendazole at ten times the normal dose for two days, fenbendazol at one-and-a-half times the normal dose for five days and oxfendazol at five times the normal dose once have all demonstrated the ability to kill parasite larvae.

These drugs have an extremely wide margin of safety and have been tested at up to 40 times overdose. They are safe for use even in young, sick or debilitated animals. There are no reported adverse effects of benzimidazole parasiticides, but products containing cambendazole are not recommended for use in pregnant mares, according to the manufacturer.

Parasite resistance primarily from one group of intestinal parasites, the "small" stongyles, has been seen against benzimidazole parasiticides. Rotational programs that include other deworming agents are therefore commonly recommended for optimum control of internal parasites in the horse.

Benzimidazoles have little or no effectiveness against tapeworms, bots or parasites of the horse's skin. Combinations of benzimidazol parasiticides and organophosphate dewormers are available for the control of bots, a parasite of the horse's stomach (see Dewormers, p. 80).

Benzimidazoles also have some antifungal activity. Consequently, they are used by some veterinarians to make antifungal preparations that may be applied to the skin of affected horses.

BENZOCAINE
Benzocaine is a local anesthetic, chemically similar to lidocaine or mepivicaine (see Lidocaine, p. 125, and Mepivicaine, p. 129). Benzocaine is a common ingredient in ointments sold over-the-counter and applied to the skin in man. Its anesthetic action helps relieve pain associated with surface ulcers and healing wounds.

Precautions
Benzocaine is considered a forbidden substance by most organizations that oversee competitions. Benzocaine is used in the preparation of some coolant gels that are applied to the horse's limbs (see Coolant Gel, p. 69). Theoretically, if benzocaine were to be absorbed by the horse's body through an open wound, the horse could test positive on drug tests for forbidden substances.

BENZYL ALCOHOL
Benzyl alcohol is normally applied to the skin of the horse. It can be used to help relieve itching and is mildly effective at controlling the growth of bacteria (see Alcohol, p. 33). Benzyl alcohol is contained in some over-the-counter wound preparations for the horse (see Wound Treatments, p. 196).

BETA-CAROTENE
Beta-carotene is the substance in the diet from which vitamin A is

formed (see Vitamin A, p. 189).

An injectable preparation of beta-carotene has been promoted as an aid in improving the reproductive efficiency of mares. There is no indication that it actually does so.

BETADINE® (see Povidone-Iodine)

BETAMETHASONE (Celestone Soluspan®)
Betamethasone is a *steroidal anti-inflammatory drug*. Beta-methasone suspension is most commonly used for injection into joints to suppress signs of inflammation associated with acute and chronic arthritis.

Precautions
When betamethasone is administered into a joint, routine cleanliness procedures should be followed to help reduce the opportunity for infection. After joint injection, it is generally felt that horses should be rested for several days prior to a gradual return to normal use.

Occasional acute inflammation ("joint flare") is seen after injection of steroids into joints, resulting in heat, pain and swelling in the affected area. This effect usually disappears rapidly but it must be quickly distinguished from a joint infection, which is a serious problem.

Side Effects
Steroidal anti-inflammatory drugs such as betamethasone have been accused of speeding up joint destruction in horses in which arthritis already exists. It is a fact that in joints, corticosteroids have been demonstrated to decrease the metabolism of cartilage cells, but how far this effect extends, and how much damage it actually causes in joints is still a matter of discussion among scientists.

Considerable evidence exists stating that injection of a corticosteroid into normal joints is not harmful to the joint surfaces, although cartilage metabolism may be affected for up to sixteen weeks after injection. Some clinicians feel that betamethasone is less likely to produce adverse effects in joints than are other corticosteroids (see Corticosteroid, p. 71).

BIGELOIL® (see Liniment)

BIOSPONGE® (see Smectite)

BIOTIN
Biotin is a vitamin. It is commonly supplemented in the horse's feed to promote improved hoof quality (see Hoof Supplements, p. 112). Initial investigations done on pigs suggested that supplementation with biotin improved hoof quality in that species. Subsequently, a few studies done in the 1980s suggested that biotin could help improve the resiliency and quality of the hoof in horses.

The hoof grows from the coronary band down to the ground. Biotin is only incorporated into the hoof at the growth level, where the hoof is still live tissue. Therefore, it may be several months before any effect from biotin supplementation is seen in the horse's hoof, and unfortunately, sometimes biotin doesn't seem to help horses' feet at all.

Neither biotin toxicity nor biotin deficiency have been reported in horses.

BISMUTH COMPOUNDS (Subsalicylate, Carbonate, etc.)
Bismuth compounds are commonly used in antacids and antidiarrheal products in people. They are occasionally used for the treatment of stomach ulcers in people. They must be given frequently, six to ten times a day, to have any effect on stomach ulcers.

In horses, very large doses of bismuth compounds would have to be given regularly to have any effect in the treatment of ulcers or diarrhea. The dose of bismuth in pastes available over-the-counter is too small to have any significant effect. Therefore, their use in the horse is limited due to the time, expense and mess involved with treatment.

They are certainly not useful in the treatment of abdominal distress (*colic*) in the horse.

BLISTER
A blister is an extreme form of a *counterirritant preparation* (see Counterirritant, p. 74). When applied to the skin of the horse, these compounds cause tremendous inflammation, swelling and pain.

"Blistering" is an outdated form of treatment that has been in

existence for literally hundreds of years. It is most commonly recommended for "treatment" of tendon and ligament injury in the
horse. Most proponents of blistering assert that by creating the
tremendous inflammation in the skin, blood is brought into the area
and healing is promoted. Nothing of the sort occurs. Good studies
have shown that blistering only inflames the skin and should have
no effect on the circulation to underlying areas.

What blistering effectively does do is enforce rest in the horse. The
afflicted leg becomes so swollen and inflamed that the horse cannot
move comfortably until the inflammation has subsided. The use of
this sort of "therapy" is condemned by the American Humane
Society.

BLOODROOT (*Sanguinaria canadensis*)
Bloodroot preparations find many uses in human medicine. In lower
concentrations, bloodroot can be used as a mouthwash or in an
effort to help remove dental plaque. Sanguinarine, the primary compound food in bloodroot, appears to have antimicrobial, antifungal,
anti-inflammatory and antihistamine activity.

In horses, a product said to be useful in the treatment of skin
cancers is available (see Xxterra, p. 198). However, this product
also contains high concentrations of zinc chloride, a caustic chemical (see Zinc Chloride, p. 200). There is no evidence that
bloodroot alone has any effectiveness in the treatment of cancer.
Caustic chemicals are something that are best applied under the
direction of your veterinarian, if at all.

Comments
During the mid-1800s, topical preparations of bloodroot extracts
were used unsuccessfully for treatment of human breast tumors.

BLU-KOTE® (see Crystal Violet, Sodium Propionate)

BOLDENONE UNDECYLENATE (Equipoise®)
Boldenone undecylenate (BOWL-den-own un-dee-SIGH-len-ate) is a
long-acting injectable anabolic steroid for intramuscular (IM)
administration in horses (see Anabolic Steroid, p. 39). It has been
used in an attempt to improve the general state of weakened horses
and to help in improving appetite. It should be considered only as

an adjunct to therapy for specific disease, surgery and traumatic injury. In conditions where the drug may be effective, most horses will reportedly respond with one or two treatments.

Precautions

This drug is a controlled substance by the US Food and Drug Administration (USFDA) because of its potential for abuse by humans.

Side Effects

This drug possesses marked *androgenic effects*. Androgenic effects are those associated with stallion-like behaviors. Thus, overaggressiveness may be noted in horses given this drug. If these effects occur, they may last for up to six or eight weeks, according to the manufacturer.

Studies in mares given boldenone undecylenate show interference with normal estrous behavior ("heat"). Normal cycles eventually do resume once the drug is withdrawn; however, it may take several months (see Stanozolol, p. 175).

BORIC ACID

Boric acid is a very weak germicide that is extremely nonirritating. It is used in some preparations to wash out the eye.

Boric acid is also added to some preparations that are used on the hoof (see Hoof Dressings, p. 111). There seems to be little use for boric acid on the horse's hoof.

BOSWELLIA SERRATA (Indian Frankincense)

Like most herbal products, the uses of *Boswellia* (also known as Indian frankincense) are numerous. In people, the plant is used for osteoarthritis, rheumatism, bursitis, tendonitis, abdominal pain, asthma, sore throat, syphilis, pimples [sic] and cancer. It is also used as a stimulant, respiratory antiseptic and diuretic. In manufacturing, Indian frankincense resin oil and extracts are used in soaps, cosmetics, foods and beverages. For horses, it is a component of one preparation intended for "joint health."

There is absolutely no indication that *Boswellia* is effective for any of its uses.

BRACE
The term "brace" is a synonym for liniment (see Liniment, p. 126).

BREWER'S YEAST
Brewer's yeast is a source of B-vitamins and protein for horses. Horses obtain all the B-vitamins that they need from their diet and from synthesis of the vitamins by bacteria in the intestines. There are no reports of deficiencies or toxicities of B-vitamins in the horse, nor is there evidence of toxicity caused by supplementation with brewer's yeast. Other, less expensive protein supplements are available should this form of supplementation be desired (see Vitamin B, p. 190, and Protein, p. 163).

BURDOCK ROOT
Burdock is a stout, common weed native to Europe and northern Asia and is now widespread throughout the United States, as well. A member of the thistle family, burdock has hooked burrs that stick to clothing or animal fur.

During the Middle Ages, burdock was valued for treating a whole variety of ailments. English herbalists used burdock root for boils, scurvy (a disease caused by vitamin C deficiency, leading to bleeding, gum disease and weakness), diabetes, and rheumatism (disorders characterized by joint discomfort and loss of mobility). Burdock also played an important role in Native American herbal medicine, and American herbalists have used the roots and seeds of this plant for two centuries.

Today, in people and in horses, orally ingested burdock root is still used for innumerable purposes, including (but not limited to) as a diuretic, "blood purifier," antimicrobial or an anti-fever agent. There's no evidence that the plant actually works for any of its intended purposes, in people or in horses.

BUSCOPAN® (see N-Butylscopolammonium Bromide)

"BUTE" (see Phenylbutazone)

BUTORPHANOL (Torbugesic®)
Butorphanol (bue-TOR-fan-ol) is an *analgesic* (a pain-relieving

agent) for the horse. It comes as a sterile solution that is most commonly used intravenously (IV). Butorphanol has been shown to be effective for the relief of pain arising from colic in experimental situations, with relief lasting up to four hours.

Butorphanol is not as effective as the drugs xylazine or detomodine at relieving abdominal pain, however (see Xylazine, p. 198, and Detomodine, p. 78).

The sedative effects of butorphanol are not as profound as xylazine or detomodine, either. This is sometimes a good thing. For example, horses receiving large doses of these drugs to control pain may have trouble keeping their balance; so, to decrease the sedative side effects, butorphanol is sometimes combined with them to provide increased analgesic effects.

Clinical experience suggests that this combination of drugs also tends to reduce the horse's reaction to external stimuli when compared with the sedative effects of xylazine or detomodine alone. As such, "cocktails" of butorphanol and other drugs may be given when painful or unpleasant procedures are performed on horses.

Precautions
As with other tranquilizers, care should be used if working around horses that are under the effects of this drug. Horses are still able to react to external stimuli when they are tranquilized. There are no controlled studies on the use of butorphanol in breeding horses, weanlings or foals.

Side Effects
Toxic effects of butorphanol are not seen until the dosage is exceeded by twenty times. Mild sedation is seen in some horses following administration. The most commonly seen side effect is mild incoordination or stumbling, which can last for up to ten minutes. Occasionally, this incoordination can be more pronounced.

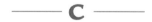

C

CACOCOPPER (CaCo-Iron-Copper)
Solutions containing the minerals calcium, cobalt and copper, plus or minus iron, have found some popularity as treatments to boost

appetite or to help speed recovery from disease (presumably, when recovery is deemed to be too slow). They may also be administered to improve haircoat. The products seem to be administered based on the whims of the person prescribing them, and there is essentially no evidence to indicate that they have any beneficial effect for the horse.

CALCIUM

Calcium is a mineral with many important functions in the horse's body, the most important function of which is as a structural component of bone. Calcium is also critical for normal muscle function.

Calcium levels are closely associated with levels of phosphorus, and both minerals are needed for normal bone formation (see Phosphorus, p. 152). The "balance" between levels of calcium and phosphorus (the calcium to phosphorus ratio) in the horse's diet has been extensively studied and is of great concern to many horse owners. As long as the minimum dietary requirements for both calcium and phosphorus are met, however, the balance of these minerals appears to be somewhat less important than the absolute levels of each mineral in the diet.

Calcium levels are largely controlled by vitamin D (see Vitamin D, p. 193). Control of body calcium levels is very complex. Naturally occurring incidences of excess calcium intoxication have not been reported. Alfalfa hay has high amounts of calcium in it and most horses get adequate amounts of dietary calcium. Calcium-deficient diets have been reported, although rarely. When combined with an excess of phosphorus, calcium deficiency can result in a condition called *nutritional secondary hyperparathyroidism*, a disease characterized by abnormalities in the bones and lameness. This condition is extremely rare today and was mostly seen in the nineteenth century when feeding large amounts of wheat bran, with it's high phosphorus and low calcium levels, became popular. The resulting condition was called "Big Head."

Significant amounts of calcium can be lost in the sweat of exercising horses and such losses are thought to be associated with a condition called "thumps" (*synchronous diaphragmatic flutter*). In heavily exercised horses, calcium loss is associated with interference with normal muscle function. Lactating mares, particularly draft horse mares, can also lose significant amounts of calcium in their milk. Additional dietary calcium will not prevent these conditions.

In the case of lactating mares, additional dietary calcium prior to giving birth actually tends to make it *more* likely that there will be a problem with excessive calcium loss in the milk. If either of these conditions occur, treatment with calcium-containing solutions must be given at the time they appear.

Calcium supplements or injections of calcium-containing solutions have been advocated by some people as a method of "natural" tranquilization for the horse. There is no medical evidence supporting the use of calcium for this purpose.

CAMPHOR

Camphor is a natural compound obtained by distilling the chips and leaves of the camphor tree. It has a distinct, characteristic odor.

Camphor has several weak pharmacologic properties. It is mildly effective as an antiseptic and an *anesthetic* (anti-itch) when applied to the skin. Camphor also has some counterirritant properties and is used in a variety of liniments for the horse applied to the leg or body (see Counterirritant, p. 74, and Liniment, p. 126). Camphor has no effect on inflammation in the deeper tissues over which it may be applied.

CAPSAICIN

Capsaicin is what makes hot chili peppers, such as cayenne or jalapeño, hot. Capsaicin is a component of several of the over-the-counter liniment products that are made for the horse. It is also the principal ingredient of a powder that people put in their socks to help their feet feel warm. Capsaicin has been used for a variety of conditions in people, such as nausea, back pain, itching, rheumatism and arthritis.

There is some experimental evidence to indicate that capsaicin-containing ointments can help reduce pain in some conditions in people. One study in horses concluded that the topical application of capsaicin ointment over the palmar digital nerves provided measurable pain relief for up to four hours after treatment. Capsaicin appears to bind to pain receptors in the skin. At first, this can cause discomfort; in people, the sensation is felt as itching, pricking or burning (see Counterirritant, p. 74). The mechanism for these effects is thought to be the result of selective stimulation of certain nerve fibers and release of a compound known as *substance P*, which mediates pain. After repeated applications of capsaicin, longer term pain relief may occur, possibly the result of substance P depletion. Long-term application of capsaicin may also cause deterioration of nerve fibers in the skin. If such effects also occur in horses is not known.

Precautions
Capsaicin is irritating to surface tissue. Topically, it can cause burning, stinging and redness. It is reported that about one in ten human patients who use capsaicin topically discontinue treatment because of adverse effects. No such data is available for horses, although one might imagine that a horse would eventually resent application of an irritating substance to his skin. Inhalation of capsaicin can cause coughing, breathing difficulties, nasal congestion and extreme eye irritation in people.

Capsaicin is a forbidden substance under USEF regulations.

CAPSICUM (see Capsaicin)

CAPTAN
Captan is a rose and plant fungicide that has been occasionally recommended for the treatment of fungal skin infections of the horse. Clinical experience with captan has shown it to be largely ineffective in the treatment of these conditions. If chosen for skin therapy, captan should be used with care. The drug commonly causes skin allergies and sensitivities in people. Captan has been classified as a probable human cancer-causing agent.

CARAFATE® (see Sucralfate)

CARBAZOCHROME SALICYLATE ("Kentucky Red," Adrenosem®)
Carbazochrome salicylate (car-BAY-za-chrome sa-LISS-a-late) has been tried in horses in an effort to prevent the bleeding that may occur from a horse's lungs due to heavy exercise (*exercise-induced pulmonary hemorrhage*, or "bleeding"). One manufacturer of the product has claimed that carbazochrome allegedly stops bleeding by reducing the permeability of small blood vessels (*capillaries*) in the lungs. Carbazochrome has been tested in aspirin-induced stomach lining

injury in rats, where it not only failed to stop injury to rat stomach lining, it *enhanced* the injury. Carbazochrome has also been shown to be ineffective in reducing capillary bleeding during human surgery.

There is no scientific proof of the efficacy or safety of carbazochrome, and until there is, there would seem to be little justification for race-day use.

CARBOCAINE® (see Mepivacaine)

CASTOR OIL
Castor oil is obtained from the seed of the castor bean plant. Its existence dates from the time of the ancient Egyptians. In man, castor oil can be used externally or internally. Internally, it acts as a *cathartic* (it causes diarrhea) and is used to empty the gastrointestinal tract. Externally, castor oil is used as an emollient (see Emollient, p. 90).
In the horse, castor oil is most commonly used externally and is a common component of various hoof dressings, presumably for its emollient properties (see Hoof Dressings, p. 111). Given internally, castor oil can cause severe diarrhea in horses.

CATAPLASM
The term cataplasm is a synonym for poultice (see Poultice, p. 157).

CEDARWOOD OIL (see Pine Oil)

CEFTIOFUR SODIUM (Naxcel®)
Ceftiofur sodium (CEFF-ti-o-fure SO-di-um) is the only member of the *cephalosporin group* of antibiotics that is approved for use in horses. These antibiotics, like the penicillins, disrupt and prevent the formation of the cell wall of certain bacteria. Other members of this group of antibiotics have wide usage in both human and veterinary medicine because they kill many different bacteria with few adverse effects.

Ceftiofur comes as a sterile powder. It is mixed with sterile water prior to administration by intramuscular (IM) injection. It is also given intravenously (IV) by some veterinarians. It appears to be effective by either route of administration.

Side Effects
Ceftiofur appears to be relatively safe for use in the horse at recommended doses. Occasional reports of diarrhea and colitis have been mentioned as potential side effects.

CETYL ALCOHOL
Cetyl alcohol is an ointment base that has wide use in the manufacture of cosmetic creams and lotions. It helps ointments retain their consistency and makes human skin feel smooth. Cetyl alcohol is a component of various hoof dressings (see Hoof Dressings, p. 111).

CETYL MYRISTOLEATE (Cetyl-M)
Cetyl myristoleate is another supplement that is promoted for the treatment and prevention of arthritis. The material is synthesized from cetyl alcohol and myristoleic acid. The rationale for its use in osteoarthritis comes from the theory that cetyl myristoleate may inhibit some metabolic pathways of a chemical important in inflammation, and therefore decrease production of some inflammatory substances by the body.

There is no good clinical evidence to support use of this product in horses or people at this time.

CHAMOMILE
The medicinal use of chamomile dates back thousands of years to the ancient Egyptians, Romans and Greeks. The tiny flowers of German chamomile have white collars circling raised, cone-shaped, yellow centers and are less than an inch wide, growing on long, thin, light green stems. The flowers look like little daisies. Sometimes chamomile grows wild and close to the ground, but you can also find it bordering herb gardens.

There are actually two plants known as chamomile: the more popular German chamomile (*Matricaria recutita*) and Roman—or English—chamomile (*Chamaemelum nobile*). Both are members of the plant family that includes ragweed and echinacea. As with most herbal preparations, both have been used for a wide number of conditions in humans, including calming frayed nerves, treating various digestive disorders, relieving muscle spasms and treating a range of skin conditions and mild infections.

A few studies in some animal species (but not horses) have suggested that German chamomile may help reduce inflammation, speed wound healing, reduce muscle spasms and serve as a mild sedative to help with sleep. Laboratory studies have also suggested that chamomile may fight against a variety of infections. In Europe, chamomile is commonly used as a digestive aid, to treat mild skin conditions, menstrual cramps, insomnia and relieve tension. The crushed, dried plant flowers also make a tasty tea.

Precautions
Chamomile can cause allergic reactions in people, although such problems are unreported in animals.

CHARCOAL
Charcoal is almost pure carbon. It is the residue of burning wood in the presence of air. Charcoal is generally treated by a number of chemical processes to increase its ability to adsorb (attract and retain material on its surface) various substances. This process is referred to as *activation*. Activated charcoal is most commonly given orally, to help absorb toxins after poisonings. Charcoal has no recognized value in the treatment of diarrhea, although it has also been used for that.

Charcoal is also available in an over-the-counter wound preparation for horses (see Wound Treatments, p. 196). There is no obvious reason why charcoal might be of benefit for treating wounds.

CHASTE BERRY (Chasteberry, Vitex Agnus-Castus)
In human females, chaste berry has been used as a treatment for premenstrual syndrome and cyclical breast discomfort. Chaste berry has been suggested as a treatment for *equine pituitary pars intermedia dysfunction (Equine Cushing's Disease—ECD)* because the fruit and seeds of the plant contain oils that appear to help the action of *dopamine*, a neurotransmitter. This mechanism of action would mirror that of the drug pergolide (see Pergolide, p. 148), although, as with all herbal products, it would be difficult to administer a consistent dose.

In horses, there is a report of chaste berry being effective for the treatment of Equine Cushing's Disease in a lay horse publication. However, one well-conducted study at the University of Pennsylvania concluded that chaste berry was not effective at treating Equine Cushing's Disease. Its use in this regard is currently being studied in the United Kingdom.

Comments
The name of the plant is due to the fact that historians say that monks chewed chaste tree parts to make it easier to maintain their celibacy.

CHELATED MINERALS
Some minerals are metallic elements, such as zinc, iron or magnesium. To *chelate* means to bind a metal element to another substance. In the case of minerals, they are often bound to amino acids, the building blocks of proteins (see Amino Acid, p. 37).

Manufacturers claim that chelated minerals are absorbed more quickly by the body than are nonchelated minerals. In fact, chelated minerals are rapidly separated from the amino acids in the stomach and intestines and are then absorbed just like nonchelated minerals. There is certainly no evidence that shows that chelated minerals are absorbed any better than nonchelated minerals. Most horses don't need mineral supplementation anyway (see Mineral, p. 134).

CHLORAMPHENICOL
Chloramphenicol is an antibiotic that is rarely used in horses but can be effective for certain infectious conditions. It inhibits bacterial protein synthesis, which keeps the bacteria from growing. In horses, it is most commonly given orally and is available in pill or capsule form. It is also available as a preparation to put in the eye to help treat infected eye injuries (*ulcers*).

Chloramphenicol is a unique drug because it has a tremendous ability to penetrate areas of the body that are not readily penetrated by other drugs, such as the chest cavity, the eye and the spinal canal. Unfortunately, for it to be effective when given orally, it is recommended that it be administered four times a day.

Precautions
In humans, chloramphenicol is rarely used because it can cause the body to stop producing red blood cells (*aplastic anemia*). (Aplastic anemia has *not* been seen in animals receiving chloramphenicol.)

63

This bad effect is not related to the dose of the drug—*any* amount of chloramphenicol, even simply exposure to the skin, can be dangerous to people who are susceptible to this effect. It has been estimated that between one in 40,000 to one in 200,000 people may be adversely affected by chloramphenicol. Because of this, the use of chloramphenicol is prohibited in animals intended for food.

Thus, chloramphenicol should be handled carefully. Latex gloves should be worn while handling the drug and care should be taken not to breathe dust from the drug or to get it in your mouth. Many people choose to wear protective face masks while giving the drug. It is quite bitter and horses do not eat it readily, so if chloramphenicol pills are used, they are usually given with a balling gun or dosing syringe, which can be quite messy. Prepared paste formulations of chloramphenicol may be obtained from licensed compounding pharmacies.

Chloramphenicol does have an effect on the enzymes of the liver. It can delay the metabolism of certain substances by the liver. Therefore, it should be employed with caution when used with other drugs that are processed by the liver, such as some anesthetic or anticonvulsant agents.

Chloramphenicol should not be administered prior to giving *barbiturate anesthetic agents* (which are commonly used to begin anesthesia in the horse). It is also recommended that the simultaneous use of chloramphenicol and *immunizing agents* (vaccines) be avoided.

Side Effects
Adverse reactions to chloramphenicol do not occur very often. In practically all respects, the drug is free of bad effects on the gastrointestinal and nervous systems. It does not seem to be associated with allergic reactions, either.

Chloramphenicol should theoretically not be used with penicillin-type drugs. Penicillins work only on growing bacteria and chloramphenicol interferes with the growth of bacteria (it does not kill them directly).

CHLORHEXIDINE (Nolvasan®, Chlorhexiderm®, Chlorasan®, Virosan®, Solvahex®)
Chlorhexidine is a disinfectant and antiseptic. Its uses are similar to povidone-iodine (see Povidone-Iodine, p. 158). When compared

with povidone-iodine, cleansing the skin with chlorhexidine causes a more immediate reduction in surface bacteria and has a longer residual action. However, experimentally chlorhexidine has been shown to slow wound healing if it is not completely rinsed from a wound in which it is used as a cleaning agent. It comes as a solution and as a solution containing soap; there is also a chlorhexidine ointment available for the treatment of wounds of the horse.

CHLOROXYLENOL

Chloroxylenol (chlor-o-ZIE-len-ol) is a derivative of coal tar oil. Chloroxylenol and related products are primarily used to preserve wood. It is found in a commonly used liniment for the horse (see Liniment, p. 126) and is of no known therapeutic value.

CHONDROITIN SULFATE (Cosequin®, Flex-Free®, etc.)

Chondroitin sulfate (CS) is an oral supplement for the horse. It is most commonly recommended for treatment of arthritis and other conditions involving joints. Chondroitin sulfate is one of a variety of substances, called *glycosaminoglycans*, that are found in normal horse joints. They are structural components of joint cartilage and connective tissues and help form the matrix that exists around cartilage cells. Most CS fed to horses is obtained from the bovine trachea.

Whether providing chondroitin sulfate in the horse's feed makes any difference in the horse is another question. Although individual studies may suggest that the product is helpful, taken as a whole, studies have largely failed to show significant benefit from chondroitin sulfate supplementation in any species. The largest study to date, in humans, failed to show the benefit of the CS supplementation for osteoarthritis of the human knee.

Due to its large molecular size, it is unlikely that the product is well-absorbed by the horse's intestines; good studies indicate that small amounts of CS may cross the upper intestine intact, but in the distal GI tract the molecule is effectively degraded, presumably by the enzymes in the intestinal flora. There is no evidence at this time to indicate that supplementation of CS products has any protective effect on joint cartilage, any anti-inflammatory effect or any lubricant effect in arthritic joints in the horse. Nor are reports of beneficial effects in horses supported by the preponderance of scientific studies at this point in time.

If it were to be effective, chondroitin sulfate should act in a similar manner as polysulfated glycosaminoglycan (see Polysulfated Glycosaminoglycan, p. 155). While the scientific evidence overall is not supportive, some veterinarians have reported beneficial effects in the treatment of arthritis with these products and they are widely promoted and used.

No adverse side effects have been reported from the use of chondroitin sulfate products in the horse.

CHROMIUM

The trace mineral chromium has received some publicity as being helpful in the control of appetite and diabetes in people. As such, it has been advocated for use in obese horses and in those with purported insulin sensitivity.

Unfortunately, recent research suggest that chromium might not be as effective for helping to treat type 2 diabetes as was previously thought. New research in an obese, Western population suggests that chromium is *not* effective for improving diabetes control in humans, whereas previous research suggested significant benefit. It turns out that the largest previous trial included patients from China, where chromium deficiency is more likely.

Chromium supplementation might only help your horse if he is chromium deficient (a condition that has never been described in horses). If there's no recognizable improvement within a few weeks of using chromium, then it probably won't help at all.

CIMETIDINE (Tagamet®)

Cimetidine is a specific type of histamine antagonist (*antihistamine*) that is occasionally used in the horse for the treatment of stomach ulcers. It has also been reported to be occasionally useful for the treatment of a specific type of melanoma (a type of skin cancer).

Cimetidine is supplied as a tablet for oral administration. The drug is quite safe and is effective for the treatment of stomach ulcers, although other drugs, including ranitidine and omeprazole, have come to be favored for treatment of this condition by many veterinarians (see Ranitidine, p. 166, and Omeprazole, p. 142).

No significant side effects have been reported from the use of cimetidine in horses.

CISPLATIN

Cisplatin is a platinum-based chemotherapy drug used in the treatment of some types of cancer. It was first discovered in the 1800s, but its anticancer properties weren't discovered until the mid-1960s, and then by accident. Cisplatin works by damaging the DNA of cancer cells, making it impossible for them to reproduce.

In horses, cisplatin, usually suspended in an oil base, has found its widest use in the treatment of two kinds of equine skin tumors: *sarcoids* and *squamous cell carcinomas*. Success rates of up to 78 percent have been reported for the use of cisplatin in the treatment of equine sarcoids.

Side Effects

Cisplatin has a number of side effects in people, including kidney and nerve damage, nausea and vomiting, so its use must be restricted to licensed veterinarians.

CINNAMON

The spice cinnamon, obtained from the dried bark of a tree, has been investigated as an aid to controlling blood sugar (*glucose*) and fats (*serum lipids*) in people and rats with type 2 diabetes. As such, it has been promoted as an aid in controlling insulin sensitivity in horses. There are no studies to indicate that cinnamon is effective in horses for such a purpose, and, indeed, the entire area of insulin sensitivity is not well-understood in horses. Nevertheless, cinnamon would be expected to be harmless for such purposes, and perhaps even tasty.

CLEAVERS

Cleavers grow in wet areas of Great Britain, Europe, Asia and North America. Small prickles grow on the leaves of cleavers, causing it to have a sticky feeling and giving it its name.

The leaves and flowers of cleavers are used orally as a diuretic, a mild astringent, for urinary problems, psoriasis and for enlarged lymph nodes. It can also be applied topically, where it's used for ulcers, festering glands and skin rashes.

There is no scientific information to suggest that the product has any medicinal effect or health benefit whatsoever.

CLENBUTEROL (VENTIPULMIN®)

Clenbuterol (clen-BUE-ter-ol) is a *bronchodilator* for oral administration in the horse. Bronchodilators are sometimes used in the management of airway problems, including *chronic obstructive pulmonary disease (COPD)*. By dilating the small air passages in the lungs (*bronchioles*), air can theoretically move in and out of the lungs more easily, making it less difficult for affected horses to breathe.

Some people have used clenbuterol in an effort to improve performance. There's no evidence that it does so, and the drug is easily detectable on drug screens. Furthermore, chronic use of clenbuterol has been shown to decrease aerobic performance in horses.

CLIOQUINOL

Clioquinol has been occasionally recommended for treatment of diarrhea of unknown causes in the horse. Topically, clioquinol has been used to treat skin infections in people. It was once available as a large pill (*bolus*) for oral administration in the horse (Rheaform®), but that product is no longer available in such a preparation. However, the drug can be obtained from licensed compounding pharmacies.

It is not known why clioquinol helps horses with diarrhea of undetermined origin. Many horses that respond to clioquinol therapy will resume diarrhea once treatment is stopped.

CLOPROSTENOL (see Prostaglandins and the Reproductive Cycle of the Mare)

COCONUT OIL

Coconut oil is obtained by pressing coconuts seeds. It has no known pharmaceutical properties, but it smells good. It is a component of a variety of hoof dressings for the horse (see Hoof Dressings, p. 111), and as an oil, it might help reduce water evaporation from the hoof wall.

COD LIVER OIL
Cod liver oil comes from steam-cooking the liver of the codfish. Cod liver oil is made up primarily of oils, but it also contains high levels of vitamins A and D and iodine. In people, it is used primarily as a vitamin supplement. Cod liver oil is not typically used externally in people.

In horses, cod liver oil is a component of some hoof dressings. What effect cod liver oil would have on horse's hoof is unknown, although because it is an oil it may have some emollient effects (see Emollient, p. 90, and Hoof Dressings, p. 111). Hoof tissue cannot use the vitamins found in cod liver oil because the tissue is already dead.

COLLOIDAL SILVER
Colloidal silver is inorganic silver in a suspending agent. It has been promoted for myriad uses in people and horses. Colloidal silver products were once available as over-the-counter products. Silver itself is a germicidal agent.

Many products are far safer and more effective than colloidal silver. Silver has no known physiological function and is not an essential mineral supplement, contrary to some promoters' claims. In 1997, the US Food and Drug Administration (USFDA) issued a final ruling indicating that colloidal silver drug products were not considered safe (among other problems, they can cause a permanent discoloring of the skin, neurological deficits, diffuse silver deposition in internal organs and renal damage) or effective. Colloidal silver products marketed for medical purposes or promoted for unsubstantiated uses are considered misbranded.

COOLANT GEL
Many attractively colored gels are available to put on the legs of the horse. These are usually sold over-the-counter and are purported to provide a cooling and anti-inflammatory effect on the limbs. They are generally used to treat what are perceived by the owner to be minor swellings or strains of the various joints, ligaments or tendons.

Coolant gels generally contain one or more of the following ingredients: menthol, camphor, thymol, witch hazel, eucalyptus oil, magnesium sulfate or other salts and various alcohols (see Camphor,

p. 58, Menthol, p. 129, Thymol, p. 183, Witch Hazel, p. 195, and Eucalyptus Oil, p. 95). In man, such ingredients are commonly used as mild counterirritants and antiseptics (see Counterirritant, p. 74). They have a very pleasant, volatile smell and they evaporate quickly. Evaporation of substances from the skin gives a cooling sensation. What, if any, effect coolant gels have on underlying tissues is unknown, at best. These products are certainly not therapeutic for more severe injuries.

Some coolant gel products contain benzocaine, a local anesthetic agent (see Benzocaine, p. 50). Care should be taken in using these products so as to avoid causing the horse to test positively for drug use in competition.

COPPER

Copper is a trace mineral (see Trace Mineral, p. 185). It is an essential part of many of the systems of the horse's body. Copper is involved in blood production, bone production and skin pigmentation, to name but a few of its functions. Copper is also important for normal function of some of the enzyme systems of the horse's body. Relationships exist between levels of copper and zinc, as well as levels of copper and molybdenum. Copper is also important for the normal absorption of iron (see Zinc, p. 200, and Iron, p. 118).

Most horse diets have adequate levels of copper and copper deficiencies are virtually unheard of in adult horses. However, it was suggested by some researchers in the 1980s that increasing levels of dietary copper in young horses may be useful in helping to prevent the occurrence of *osteochondrosis*, a disease that results in abnormal cartilage development in growing foals; hence, it found widespread use for a time.

Copper supplementation has also been recommended for the treatment of loss of skin pigment (*vitiligo*) that occurs in some horses, although there are no reports that copper supplementation has been a successful treatment for this condition.

COPPER NAPTHENATE (Kopertox®)

Copper napthenate is the main ingredient in a number of preparations for the treatment of *thrush*, an infectious condition of the horse's hoof. It is a caustic chemical that dries the hoof tissue and destroys the infectious agents. As such, it appears to be an effective treatment for controlling thrush.

Precautions
Contact with sensitive skin tissues should be avoided.

COPPER SULFATE
Copper sulfate is a chemical found in a number of preparations sold over-the-counter for wound treatment in the horse (see Wound Treatments, p. 196). Copper sulfate is a caustic chemical. It causes local tissue destruction. As a wound treatment, copper sulfate causes a hard scab to form on tissue. It causes surface proteins to come out of solution (to *precipitate*).

Copper sulfate does kill bacteria directly, but the formation of a chemical scab on healing tissue is not necessarily a good thing. In fact, the growth of bacteria may even be favored underneath the protection of the chemically caused scab.

The treatment of wounds with harsh caustic substances is generally not recommended. The rationale for inducing a chemical burn onto healing tissue is difficult to grasp.

CORTICOSTEROID
Corticosteroids are a group of hormones that are produced by the two small adrenal glands, one of which lies next to each kidney of the horse. These hormones have many extremely important functions in the horse's body.

Various synthetic hormones have been made in an attempt to help reproduce the beneficial effects of corticosteroids. These drugs are a part of medical therapy for many conditions. The most important effects of the corticosteroids in medicine are anti-inflammatory. Used correctly, corticosteroids are safe and effective agents for reducing inflammation of a variety of tissues and are very useful in combating allergic reactions. Various corticosteroid preparations are given intravenously (IV), in the muscle (IM), orally, into joints and on the surface of the body, as well as both on and in the eye. The drugs are also used in the treatment of early stages of shock. Animals that receive corticosteroid therapy seem to feel better immediately.

Many types of corticosteroid exist (see Betamethasone, p. 51, Dexamethasone, p. 81, Prednisone/Prednisolone, p. 159, and

Triamcinolone, p. 185). There are differences in potency and duration of action among the various agents, but selection of various corticosteroid drugs is largely a matter of the experience of the veterinarian and the cost of the drug. There is no consensus in the veterinary community as to which steroid is the "best" for use in any one condition.

It is important to realize that corticosteroids are not a cure for any disease process. Their anti-inflammatory effects can quiet a variety of inflammatory conditions and this is certainly useful, but relief is frequently only temporary. In the treatment of conditions such as arthritis, for example, corticosteroids can help alleviate inflammation of the joint. However, the arthritis is not cured by the treatment. Similarly, corticosteroids can control the abnormal responses seen with allergic reactions (such as *hives*) but they do not desensitize the horse to whatever it is that he is allergic to.

Precautions
Corticosteroid drugs should be used very carefully in the face of infection. While corticosteroid products are good agents for the relief of inflammation, inflammation is an important and necessary response of the body to help combat infection. If the inflammatory response is suppressed, infection may be able to spread more easily. Similarly, while corticosteroid agents suppress the immune system when it's out of control (that's why, for example, they help control allergies), this effect is not at all good when the body is trying to fight off an infection. The body needs a fully functioning immune system to help combat disease-producing agents. For the same reasons, corticosteroids should not be given at the same time as vaccines, so as to avoid impeding the normal immune response to vaccination.

Corticosteroid preparations should never be used to treat an eye that has an ulcer in its surface. Ulcers are disruptions in the surface of the *cornea* (the covering of the eye) that most commonly occur from trauma to the eye. Corticosteroids retard or prevent healing on the ulcerated surface of the eye.

Corticosteroid ointments can be applied to skin wounds to help control the growth of granulation tissue (see Wound Treatments, p. 196). A few days after the occurrence of a wound on the skin, corticosteroid ointments applied to the wound surface have no adverse effect on healing.

Because corticosteroids can induce labor in some species, some people have advised caution in giving corticosteroids to mares that are late in their pregnancies. However, in scientific studies, pregnant mares have not been shown to abort their fetuses when given corticosteroids.

Side Effects

It is generally accepted in medicine that to prevent negative effects of corticosteroids—or of any drug—the drugs should be used at the lowest effective dose possible for the shortest period of time necessary. In the body, naturally occurring levels of corticosteroid-like substances are carefully controlled by a complex mechanism. Corticosteroids are synthetic drugs that mimic the effects of the naturally occurring substances. If the drugs are administered regularly and in high enough doses, the body may not feel the need to produce its own corticosteroids, relying instead on the drug from the outside. This is loosely referred to as *drug dependence*. Once the drug is removed, then, the body may not be ready to produce the required "natural" amounts of the hormone. This can cause serious health problems. For this reason, it is commonly recommended in most species that corticosteroids be withdrawn from the body slowly, with a decreasing dosage over a period of time.

Prolonged corticosteroid therapy in dogs or humans also commonly produces a whole host of other side effects, such as weight gain, increased appetite, increased thirst, increased urination, gastrointestinal ulceration and tissue wasting. For some reason, however, horses seem to be particularly insensitive to the negative effects of corticosteroids and of drug dependence—they seem to tolerate relatively large doses of these drugs for prolonged periods of time with few adverse side effects and little need for slow withdrawal. Many veterinarians prefer, however, to slowly withdraw horses from corticosteroid therapy just in case negative effects might be seen.

In horses, two significant side effects of corticosteroid drugs *are* reported. *Laminitis* ("founder") is a serious condition affecting the hoof of the horse. Although no direct causal link has been established, the use of corticosteroid drugs has occasionally been associated with the onset of laminitis. High doses and prolonged use of longer-acting systemic corticosteroid products are reportedly risk factors for causing laminitis. It is generally considered that corticosteroids should not be used in the treatment of laminitis because they help decrease the flow of blood to the hoof.

Steroidal anti-inflammatory drugs have also been accused of accelerating joint destruction in horses, especially those that have pre-existing arthritis. Some people have accepted this as fact. The medical studies are far from clear, however. It is true that corticosteroids have the effect of impeding normal tissue metabolism. In a joint, this effect would tend to retard or prevent the normal processes, including the process of repair of damaged tissue. Theoretically, then, if the joint is prevented from repairing itself, destruction of the joint could continue without interference, leading to the so-called *steroid arthropathy*.

However, steroid arthropathies have rarely been described in horses. Certainly, the negative side effects of corticosteroid injections should be considered if they are to be given into arthritic joints, but not all joints injected with corticosteroids will develop steroid arthropathies and many arthritic joints benefit from the relief of inflammation, even if only temporarily. There is some good evidence that the drugs, when used appropriately, actually protect joint cartilage.

There is little experimental information regarding the effects of injection of corticosteroidal anti-inflammatory agents into previously damaged or arthritic joints. Considerable evidence exists showing that injection of steroids into normal joints is not harmful. The actual effects of corticosteroid injection into joints is the cause of much discussion in the veterinary community.

CORTISONE

Cortisone is a generic term that is used to describe a variety of drugs referred to as corticosteroids (see Corticosteroid, p. 71). However, there is no drug used in the horse by the name of "cortisone."

COUNTERIRRITANT

A counterirritant is a substance that, when applied to the surface of the skin, produces mild irritation and inflammation. Counterirritant effects are caused primarily by local blood vessel dilation, which, in humans, produces a sensation of heat, discomfort and sometimes itching. When the irritation is severe, these agents cause damage to surface capillaries. Plasma leaking from damaged capillaries results in the formation of blisters (see Blister, p. 52).

The concept of counterirritation is very old, probably even prehistoric. Hundreds of years ago, it was thought that inflammation could not exist in two places at one time. As a result, counterirritation was developed as a method of inciting inflammation in one area so as to relieve it in another. This concept, of course, is not true; inflammation can exist simultaneously in many areas.

In humans, counterirritants are commonly applied to the skin to help relieve muscle soreness and stiffness. The sensation of heat produced by the irritation caused by these agents does seem to help relieve minor stiffness and soreness in some cases. The reason for this effect is poorly understood.

Many counterirritant products are available for use in the horse. Whether horses have the same response to counterirritant therapy as do humans is pure speculation. What, if any, effect they have in the horse is unknown. This fact has not, of course, limited their use.

CREATINE
Creatine is a substance that normally is found within the cells of the horse's body. Creatine's role within the cell is to rapidly make *ATP* (energy) available during times of high energy consumption, such as exercise.

As such, creatine has been promoted as a supplement for horses engaging in heavy exercise. In the only large study to date, twelve purebred Arabian horses were submitted to aerobic training for 90 days, with and without 75 grams daily creatine supplementation, and then evaluated. It was not possible to show any beneficial effect from creatine on the skeletal muscle characteristics examined.

Horses, according to one expert in *New Scientist* magazine, are already endowed with a "near perfect balance between lungs, heart and muscle. Unlike human athletes, horses simply don't have much room for improvement" (Budiansky 1996).

CREOSOTE
Creosote is a mixture of volatile chemicals (*phenols*) that is obtained from wood tar. One of its main components is guaiacol (see Guaiacol, p. 110).

Creosote has very weak antiseptic properties. It has been used in steam inhalers as an expectorant (see Expectorant, p. 96). It is also occasionally used as a disinfectant (see Disinfectant, p. 88).

Creosote was previously also used as a wood preservative. It has been used to paint fences to keep horses from eating them, since it has a bitter taste. Creosote, however, is very toxic, and horses eating creosote-treated wood can conceivably be poisoned, so it is now largely unavailable for that purpose. Creosote is a component of an over-the-counter poultice for use in horses, possibly because it is a disinfectant. There are no other known medicinal properties of creosote that would explain why it would be included in such a preparation.

CRESOL
Cresol is obtained from coal tar or crude oil. It is similar to phenol in its medicinal qualities (see Phenol, p. 150). Cresol has disinfectant and antiseptic properties, but it is of very low potency. It is sometimes used to wash floors. Cresol is a component of an over-the-counter hoof dressing (see Hoof Dressings, p. 111).

CRYSTAL VIOLET ("Blue Lotion," Blu-Kote®)
Crystal violet (also known as gentian violet, methyl violet and by many other names) is a dye that is used in the treatment of surface wounds of the horse (see Wound Treatments, p. 196). Crystal violet is a weak antifungal and antibacterial agent that's typically prepared as a solution in water for application to the horse's skin. Although crystal violet is effective at killing surface bacteria and fungi, it is messy, and it turns the horse purple where it is applied, usually staining the hands and clothes of the owner at the same time. Crystal violet has also been used to treat burns in people.

Comments
Engineering students of Queen's University, Kingston, Ontario, Canada, traditionally use crystal violet to dye their whole bodies purple in preparation for homecoming celebrations. In human forensic medicine, crystal violet was used to develop fingerprints.

CYPROHEPTADINE
Cyproheptadine (sigh-pro-HEPT-a-deen) is an antihistamine that has been used in people to treat irritated, itchy, watery eyes; sneez-

ing; and runny nose caused by allergies, hay fever, and the common cold. It has also been used to relieve the itching of insect bites, bee stings, poison ivy and poison oak.

In horses, cyproheptadine has typically been prescribed to treat horses with head shaking from unknown causes (*idopathic head shaking*), and Equine Cushing's Disease (ECD). It has been shown to be moderately effective for the treatment of head shaking. In the treatment of Equine Cushing's Disease, cyproheptadine has been shown to be less effective than pergolide in some studies (see Pergolide, p. 148). The use of pergolide and cyproheptadine together has been described for the treatment of the Disease.

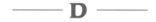

D

DANDELION

Hundreds of species of dandelion grow in the temperate regions of Europe, Asia and North America. Dandelion is a hardy, variable perennial that can grow to a height of nearly 12 inches. Dandelions have deeply notched, toothy, spatula-like leaves that are shiny and hairless. A head of bright yellow flowers caps the stems. The name of the plant apparently comes from the old French for "lion tooth" (*dent de lion*), which describes the plant's sharply indented leaves.

Dandelion can act as a mild diuretic that increases urine production by promoting the excretion of salts and water from the kidney. Although there is essentially no good evidence to support it, dandelion is used for a wide range of conditions in people, such as poor digestion, liver disorders and high blood pressure. Dandelion is also a source of potassium. The leaves can be used to make salads and wine.

Fresh or dried dandelion plants may also be used as a mild appetite stimulant and to help treat upset stomachs. The root of the dandelion plant is believed to have mild laxative effects and is often used to improve digestion. Some preliminary animal studies suggest that dandelion may help normalize blood sugar levels in diabetic mice. However, not all animal studies have had the same positive effect on blood sugar.

Comments
The late Varro Tyler, PhD, author of several popular texts on

medicinal herbs in human medicine, noted that the culinary uses of dandelion far outweigh the medicinal ones.

DESLORELIN

Deslorelin helps augment the effect of the steroid hormone *GnRH (gonadotropin releasing hormone)* in mares (see GnRH, p. 108). Normally, GnRH is released in pulses throughout the estrous ("heat") cycle. As the time of ovulation nears, the frequency of these pulses increases, which causes the release of another hormone, *luteinizing hormone (LH)*. LH then causes ovulation to occur.

Deslorelin working in a manner similar to *human chorionic gonadotropin*, or *HCG* (see Human Chorionic Gonadotropin, p. 112), by mimicking the action of LH. However, it works without causing antibodies to be produced against it, problems that have been associated with loss of effectiveness for HCG.

Deslorelin was formerly marketed as Ovuplant® in the US, as an implant to induce ovulation in mares. It was pulled from the market in the US because mares receiving the implant sometimes had extended periods where they did not come back into heat. It is still available from Canada or compounding pharmacists.

DETOMODINE (Dormosedan®)

Detomodine is a sedative and analgesic agent. It is from the same class of drugs as xylazine and romifidine (see Xylazine, p. 198, and Romifidine, p. 168). Detomodine comes as a sterile solution for intramuscular (IM) or intravenous (IV) injection.

When compared to xylazine, the sedative effects of detomodine are two to three times as long-lasting, depending on the dose. It also produces a deeper, more profound sedation than does xylazine. Horses usually stand very still, with their heads low to the ground, after they have received an injection of detomodine. These qualities can be useful during minor surgical procedures, where redosing of drugs may be inconvenient or impractical.

As an analgesic, detomodine is extremely effective for the control of abdominal pain (*colic*). The length of time that pain relief lasts depends on the dose. Detomodine appears to be able to control most types of severe colic pain. Because of this, it may mask pain signs that would indicate that a colic requires surgery to correct the problem. A thorough evaluation of the horse is imperative while pain control with detomodine is maintained.

Detomodine is also used to cause chemical ejaculation in stallions that may have difficulty being collected under normal circumstances.

Detomodine is safe at five to ten times normal doses.

Precautions

Detomodine should not be used in horses with abnormal heart rhythms, heart insufficiencies, respiratory disease or chronic kidney failure. The effects of detomodine on breeding horses and fetuses have not been studied.

Caution should always be used when working around any sedated horse. Even though deeply sedated, some horses may still respond to external stimuli. Routine safety precautions should always be used around horses sedated with detomodine or any other drug.

Detomodine use is forbidden in show horses. After administration of detomodine, drug residues can be detected for up to 60 days. The test does not identify levels of the drug, only its presence.

Side Effects

After dosage with detomodine, it is common to observe a heart rhythm abnormality known as *second degree A-V (atrio-ventricular) block*. This is best described as the heart having a pattern of regularly slowing down and then skipping a beat. This side effect is apparently not dangerous for the horse.

Sweating is also common after administration of detomodine. This is an effect of the drug on sweat glands and is not a sign of an abnormal or dangerous response.

Detomodine causes a long-term sedation that is most obviously manifested by the horse lowering his head. Sometimes swelling or passive congestion of the gums, lips or facial area may be seen if the horse's head stays down for a period of time (the circulatory system has difficulty building up enough pressure to get all the fluid out of the lowered head). Mucous discharges from the nose may be seen as well. These effects are not serious and may be relieved by elevating the head.

Urination usually occurs after recovery from detomodine sedation, usually at about 45 to 60 minutes after injection.

DEVIL'S CLAW (*Harpagophytum procumbens*)

People use devil's claw for osteoarthritis, non-specific lower back pain and many other inflammatory conditions. The root of the plant contains chemicals (*iridoid glycosides*) that have been shown to have anti-inflammatory and heart-related effects in some studies.

Preliminary evidence suggests that devil's claw extract might be inactivated by stomach acid, although the evidence is disputed. It is currently not known if the product is effective in horses.

Side Effects

In people, the most common adverse effect is diarrhea, but nausea, vomiting, and abdominal pain have also been reported. Devil's claw can cause allergic skin reactions. There is also a report of throbbing frontal headache, tinnitus (ringing of the ears), anorexia and loss of taste. Adverse reactions are unreported in horses.

Comments

The botanical name *Harpagophytum* means "hook plant" in Greek. The plant, which is native to Africa, gets its name from the appearance of its fruit, which is covered with hooks meant to attach onto animals in order to spread seeds

DEWORMERS

Many agents exist for the control of intestinal parasites in the horse. They come in one of three formulations: oral paste, liquid for administration by *nasogastric tube* (stomach tube) and powdered or pelleted for application in or on the feed.

Dozens of studies have shown that all of the above formulations appear to be equally effective in controlling intestinal parasites, assuming that: (1) the horse is given the proper dose for his weight, and (2) the horse gets the whole dose. One comparison showed that even if some wastage or loss occurs when oral pastes are given, this is probably not enough to be significant.

Occasional *nasogastric intubation* ("tube worming") is not necessary for control of internal parasites in the horse. While the stomach tube does deliver all of the medication into the horse's stomach or lower esophagus, this offers no particular advantage over oral pastes or feed-based pellets. Also, the formulations that are delivered via a tube are of no greater potency than other formulations.

Deworming products are generally quite safe and have a wide margin of safety. Many of the drugs have been tested at up to 40 times normal dose with few adverse effects. Exceptions to this were the products that contained *organophosphate chemicals* such as trichlorfon (these products are no longer commonly used). Organophosphates have occasionally been reported to cause adverse effects such as staggering or seizure at normal doses, and are not safe at twice normal doses. Moxidectin-containing products also have a narrower margin of safety than do other deworming agents. Occasional allergic reactions have also been reported in relation to deworming products, especially ivermectin. (For additional information on individual deworming products, see Ivermectin, p. 120, Moxidectin, p. 135, Benzimidazol, p. 49, Pyrantel, p. 165, and Piperazine, p. 153).

DEXAMETHASONE (Azium®, Dexameth-a-Vet®, Dexasone®)

Dexamethasone is a corticosteroid product for the control of inflammation in the horse. It is available as a sterile solution for intramuscular (IM) or intravenous (IV) injection and it can be obtained as a powder or pill for oral administration. Research has shown that the injectable product is well-absorbed when given orally, as well.

Two types of solutions of dexamethasone are available for use. *Dexamethasone sodium phosphate* is considered a rapid-onset corticosteroid. *Dexamethasone acetate* is considered to have a longer duration of action. These differences are due to the chemical configuration of the different products.

Some people feel that dexamethasone has a calming effect on horses, and thus it is occasionally used in an attempt to quiet horses prior to competitions. There is no medical evidence that the drug is effective when used in this way. The potential side effects of repeated doses of dexamethasone should also be considered before using the drug in this manner.

Precautions and Side Effects

Dexamethasone should be used with the same precautions, and has the same side effects as any of the corticosteroid agents (see Corticosteroid, p. 71). Many of the products contain label-warnings about the drug's potential to cause *laminitis*, a serious condition of the horse's feet. However, while stories of laminitis following dexamethasone administration abound, so far, no one has been able to cause laminitis in horses with dexamethasone in experimental settings.

DEXTROSE

Dextrose is a sugar and sugar provides calories. Dextrose is available as a sterile solution for intravenous (IV) administration. It is also commonly added to electrolyte supplements for oral administration in the horse.

As a practical matter, dextrose administration is rarely required for treatment of any condition of the normal horse. Dextrose solutions are probably best employed when horses are not eating normally, due to disease processes, for example. They also have some use in the treatment of shock. Still, in horses that are weak and debilitated, dextrose solutions alone are not able to meet all of the metabolic needs of the horse.

Foals do not have the same metabolic reserves as adult horses; that is, they are not very big and they have very little fat. Consequently, dextrose solutions are commonly used to help maintain energy levels in sick foals.

The oral dextrose that is provided in electrolyte preparations is in insufficient amounts to have any significant effect at the recommended dosages.

Precautions
Overuse of dextrose solutions can increase dehydration by causing water to be excreted by the kidneys. Too much sugar in the blood has to be removed from the system. That job is the kidneys' responsibility. In the process, water, as well as sodium, is lost by the horse's body.

Side Effects
There are no reported adverse side effects to dextrose at normal doses.

DIAZEPAM (Valium®)

Diazepam is a sedative agent that is rarely used in the horse. It comes as a sterile solution for intramuscular (IM) or intravenous (IV) injection.

Diazepam has little use in the horse on its own. The effects of the drug are not profound and the quality of sedation that is produced is not desirable for minor surgical procedures or for other situations where sedation is desired. However, the use of diazepam to try to calm competitive show horses has been alleged. The drug is easily detectable.

Diazepam has been used in combination with ketamine and xylazine in the horse in an effort to help smooth induction and recovery during general anesthesia (see Ketamine Hydrochloride, p. 122, and Xylazine, p. 198). Here, the drug is used for its muscle relaxant properties.

DICLOFENAC (Surpass®)

Diclofenac is one of many from the class of drugs called *nonsteroidal anti-inflammatory drugs*, although it has some unique actions that are different from similar drugs (see Nonsteroidal Anti-Inflammatory Drug, p. 141). Diclofenac works by reducing substances that cause inflammation and pain in the body. In the United States, oral preparations of diclofenac are available for people, and in some other countries, diclofenac-containing gels and creams are available to rub directly onto inflamed or sore areas.

For horses, diclofenac is available as a cream that is applied directly to the affected area, twice daily for ten days. In one study, diclofenac liposomal cream was shown to reduce lameness as graded by owners and veterinarians, regardless of the severity or duration of the clinical condition. Another study suggested that the cream may be effective for reducing subcutaneous inflammation in horses.

Urine and serum concentrations of diclofenac have been detected following topical administration of 1 percent liposomal diclofenac cream for ten days at the labeled dose and at two times and four times the labeled dose. The drug is slowly absorbed and eliminated when placed on the skin. The product should be used with caution before a competition in order to prevent an inadvertent positive drug test.

Comments

It has been reported that veterinary diclofenac use in India has caused a crash of the vulture population, with major ecological consequences. Diclofenac causes kidney failure in vultures that eat treated domestic animals.

DIMETHYLGLYCINE (DMG)

DMG is a dietary supplement present in many foods. It is supposed to increase the utilization of oxygen and decrease the production of lactic acid by the muscles during high-intensity exercise.

Several studies on DMG in people have shown that it does not have any consistent effects. The studies that have been done in horses have shown conflicting results. One study has suggested that DMG may reduce lactic acid levels in exercising horses. However, another more recent study concluded that exercising horses given DMG had no improvement in oxygen carrying by the blood—nor was there any change in lactic acid concentration in the plasma, blood or muscle in this study.

In humans, DMG has also been advocated to help improve the immune response to viral agents. This effect has not been demonstrated in horses.

In horses, DMG has most commonly been promoted as a substance to help reduce the incidence of acute or chronic *equine exertional rhabdomyolysis* (also known as "tying up," *myositis* or *azoturia*). There is no scientific evidence to suggest that DMG actually would do this. Furthermore, the mechanism by which it would exert its effect is somewhat unclear, as lactic acid production (as measured in the blood) does not appear to be a feature of rhabdomyolysis in the horse.

DIMETHYL SULFOXIDE (DMSO, Domoso®)

One of the most frequently employed and curious substances with which to treat horses is a chemical solvent containing a variety of unique and interesting properties. It has been credited—legitimately or not—with over 30 properties for the treatment of disease and is therefore used in a wide variety of applications in the horse. This substance goes by the name of dimethyl sulfoxide, abbreviated to DMSO.

DMSO is available in a gel or in a liquid form. The liquid form can be given orally, intravenously (when diluted) or applied on top of the skin; the gel is always used topically. The use of the drug is generally based on the veterinarian's experience and what he/she has read.

As a therapeutic agent, DMSO is used primarily as an anti-inflammatory. There are a variety of ways that DMSO might exert its effect as an anti-inflammatory, of which the most important seems to be the neutralization of some of the destructive substances that are produced by the process of inflammation. In addition to this, DMSO has some of the same anti-inflammatory properties as do corticosteroids (see Corticosteroids, p. 71). DMSO can be used at the same time as these drugs. DMSO will even help protect tissue from injury induced by a lack of blood (called *ischemia*—you can make your finger ischemic by putting a tight rubber band around it, for example). There are a variety of other potentially useful properties of DMSO, too. And because DMSO has such a wide array of alluring medical possibilities for treatment, it is used quite a bit in veterinary medicine in some circles.

DMSO is unique in that it can go through the skin and mucous membranes without disrupting them. Because of this property, it can be used as a carrier of other substances through the skin. When DMSO is mixed with corticosteroids, for instance, the level of the corticosteroids in the tissue is increased by a factor of three! And because it can go through the skin, people who use DMSO report tasting it after they put it on (or in) their horse.

DMSO is very volatile. When it is absorbed through the skin, it rapidly enters the circulatory system. The DMSO travels around until it reaches the lungs, at which point it exits the system and gets breathed out. Of course, the air that is breathed out travels up the back of your mouth, and that is why it can be tasted. People report that DMSO tastes like onions or garlic; although the taste may be unpleasant, it certainly isn't harmful. Horses will give off this same odor in their breath for some time after they have received significant amounts of DMSO.

The wide variety of conditions that DMSO is used to treat almost defies belief. There are reports of using it topically to treat swellings; injecting it into joints; using it systemically for muscle soreness, disease of the nervous system and treatment of colic and its associated effects; in the reproductive tract of the mare; for skin conditions; to accelerate wound healing; to prevent blood clotting; and for laminitis, to name but a few. Because of its ability to penetrate membranes, DMSO is also commonly employed to help get drugs into areas that are hard to reach, like the brain or the chest cavity. So, if it some-times seems that DMSO is being used to treat almost everything, it's because it probably is.

Unfortunately, there are no standard doses that have been gener-ated for DMSO. For most drugs, dose ranges based on half-lives and desired blood levels have been established (see p. 6). With, DMSO this is not the case. Furthermore, most of the things that DMSO is used for are outside those recommended by the manufacturer.

Finally, and importantly, no controlled studies have been done to establish how well DMSO actually works in treating most medical conditions for which it is used in the horse. As frequently as it is used, surprisingly little study has gone into its application. When it comes to DMSO and treating horses, the "cart" (frequency of use) is clearly before the "horse" (proof of effectiveness). Fortunately, and especially so considering how widely it is used, DMSO is pretty benign and has a very low toxicity. It is so safe that it can be drunk and given intravenously (although it should be diluted first to help prevent destruction of red blood cells in the blood).

DINOPROST (see Prostaglandins and the Reproductive Cycle of the Mare)

DIOCTYL SODIUM SULFOSUCCINATE (DSS)

Dioctyl sodium sulfosuccinate (di-OCT-uhl SO-di-um sul-fo-SUCK-sin-ate), or DSS, is sometimes used for the treatment of colic. It acts to reduce surface tension in the fecal mass. By doing so, DSS is sup-posed to allow water to more easily penetrate masses of fecal matter. In addition, DSS causes the intestine to secrete fluid and electrolytes. As such, it can function as a stool softener and laxative. DSS is a liq-uid that is diluted with water and given by *nasogastric intubation* (stomach tube).

DSS can also be diluted with water and given in an enema to foals for treatment of retained *meconium* (the first fecal material the foal passes).

Precautions
Theoretically, DSS should not be given at the same time as mineral oil as it has the potential to break down mineral oil into small enough

globules that it can be absorbed into the circulation. There are no reports of such a thing happening in scientific literature, however.

Side Effects
DSS has the potential to be irritating to the intestinal tract. Overdosage of DSS can create diarrhea and make horses feel quite sick. Recommended doses of DSS should probably be repeated only every 48 hours.

DIPYRONE
Dipyrone is a mild anti-inflammatory, *antipyretic* (fever controlling) and *analgesic* (pain relieving) that was once commonly used in horses (see Nonsteroidal Anti-Inflammatory Drug, p. 141). Dipyrone is chemically related to phenylbutazone and works in the same fashion (see Phenylbutazone, p. 150).

Dipyrone was once supplied as a sterile solution for intramuscular (IM), intravenous (IV) or subcutaneous administration. Dipyrone was most commonly used for the control of abdominal pain (*colic*) in the horse. However, experiments have shown that the drug is certainly not very potent.

The US Food and Drug Administration (USFDA) Center for Veterinary Medicine issued a "CVM Update" on December 6, 1995, announcing that dipyrone products had not been the subject of an approved New Animal Drug Application (NADA), and that the agency would no longer grant regulatory discretion for the marketing of these products. Currently, dipyrone is not approved for any use in animals. The use of dipyrone is considered illegal by the USFDA.

Precautions
If dipyrone is given for a prolonged period, problems with decreased white blood cells may be seen. The drug should not be used at the same time as barbiturate agents (commonly used to induce anesthesia in the horse). If given in the vein, dipyrone should be given very slowly to avoid convulsions. It should be used with care in horses with heart disease.

Side Effects
Side effects of dipyrone are similar to those of aspirin (see Aspirin, p. 43). Overdosage of dipyrone can cause seizures.

DISINFECTANT

A disinfectant is an agent that kills disease-causing microorganisms. The term is properly used when referring to killing microorganisms on inanimate objects, such as surgical instruments or the walls or floors of stalls.

DMSO (see Dimethyl Sulfoxide)

DOMPERIDONE

Domperidone was first proposed as a treatment for *fescue grass toxicity* in horses. Fescue grass can become infested with an *endophyte*. The term endophyte refers to a situation where one organism lives inside another. In this case, a fungus and grass form a relationship that is mutually beneficial and enhances the reproductive success of each.

Pregnant mares who graze on endophyte-infested fescue grass have increased gestation lengths, fail to produce milk, have increased foal and mare mortality, develop tough and thickened placentas, have weak and dysmature foals and sweat more during warm weather. Domperidone helps prevent these problems by counteracting the effects of the endophyte.

Domperidone has also been successfully used to stimulate milk production in mares that fail to produce enough milk. Between the desire to increase lactation and make sure there's no problem with the pasture grass, domperidone finds a lot of use in some circles.
It has also been investigated for use in the diagnosis of Equine Cushing's Disease (ECD).

DORMOSEDAN® (see Detomodine)

DOXYCYCLINE

Doxycycline is a tetracycline antibiotic (see Tetracycline, p. 181). It can be given orally to horses, which presents some significant treatment advantages. Doxycycline finds wide use in the treatment of Lyme disease in horses. Doxycycline has also been advocated by some veterinarians for the treatment of laminitis, due to its ability to bind an inflammatory compound (MMP-3) that has been implicated in that condition.

—— **E** ——

ECHINACEA
In people, orally administered echinacea is used for treating and preventing the common cold and other upper respiratory infections. Echinacea is also used in an effort to try to stimulate the immune system to fight a variety of other infections (although it can be argued that such stimulation would not necessarily be a good thing). The evidence for clinical trials in people is conflicting. That is, some studies show some effect in treating colds; other, high-quality trials show no effect. Most studies conclude that echinacea has no benefit in preventing colds, however.

To be fair, echinacea is inherently hard to study. The active ingredient(s) have not been identified, so no one knows why it might work. That also means that products can't be standardized, and, as a result, echinacea products intended for humans can vary significantly from product to product and even lot to lot. There are also several plant species, plant parts and preparation or extraction methods that go into echinacea products, all of which can affect the chemical makeup of the herbal product. So, insofar as using the product goes, it's a bit of therapeutic roulette.

One study has been done to see if echinacea has an effect on the immune system of the horse. In this study of eight horses, various measurements of immune system function seemed to be positively affected. The authors of the study concluded that echinacea effectively stimulated the equine immune system and behaved as a *hematinic agent* (a so-called "blood builder"). These results have not been confirmed by additional studies.

Comments
Echinacea species are native to North America and were used as traditional herbal remedies by the Great Plains Indian tribes and later adopted for medicinal use by settlers. The use of echinacea fell out of favor in the United States with the discovery of antibiotics and due to the lack of scientific data supporting its use. Its resurgence has coincided with the current interest in "alternative" medicine.

EFUDEX® (see 5-Fluorouracil)

ELECTROLYTES

Electrolyte is actually a chemical term that refers to how a substance behaves when it is put into a solution. In horses, the word electrolyte is commonly applied to a variety of *trace elements* found in sweat, most particularly the ions of sodium, potassium, calcium and chlorine.

The loss of extensive amounts of these ions via the sweat can occur in horses, particularly during endurance-type exercise. Electrolytes in the body are responsible for the transmission of the body's electrical signals; when amounts are insufficient, weakness, disorientation and abnormal muscle function can occur.

People used to take lots of electrolytes in the form of salt pills prior to exercise. Nutritionists found that this caused people to retain water and not sweat well, which is dangerous in hot weather. Horses generally don't need extra electrolytes. Even in the hottest weather, horses usually get all the electrolytes they need in their feed. However, at least one study suggests that giving horses a highly concentrated electrolyte paste prior to competition may improve endurance.

It is possible to make a horse sweat out a significant portion of his electrolytes by riding him hard in hot weather and not stopping to rest him or give him water. During a 100-mile endurance ride, for example, it's a good idea to give your horse extra electrolytes along with lots of water. Indeed, providing water, glucose and electrolytes to working endurance horses does seem to delay fatigue in these animals. Horses lose water much faster than they do electrolytes when they exercise, however, and no matter how many electrolytes you give your horse in hot weather, if you don't let him have water you're going to have some real trouble.

EMOLLIENT

Emollients are fatty substances which are generally applied to the skin or hoof of the horse. Emollients tend to make the skin feel softer because they penetrate into the surface layers of the skin (they go no deeper). They also tend to interfere with the loss of water by the skin or surface tissues.

Emollient effects are not necessarily beneficial. The retention of water and the exclusion of air that is caused by a layer of emollient may actually be favorable to the growth of bacteria that do not require oxygen (*anaerobic bacteria*). Additionally, rubbing the skin while applying emollients may actually help spread bacteria and debris.

Emollient agents are commonly used to help make various over-the-counter preparations such as hoof ointments, wound treatments and liniments (see Hoof Dressings, p. 111, Wound Treatments, p. 196, and Liniment, p. 126). Contrary to popular belief, emollients *do not* help medication penetrate the skin, nor do they help "draw out" toxic substances from below the skin.

Commonly used emollients in the horse include castor oil, cottonseed oil, glycerin, lanolin and petrolatum (see Castor Oil, p. 60, Lanolin, p. 124, and Petrolatum, p. 149).

ENROFLOXACIN (Baytril®)
Enrofloxacin (en-roe-FLOX-a-sin) is a member of a class of antibacterial agents called *fluroroquinolones*. It is a pretty new class of well-tolerated, fairly safe drugs that kill a wide number of important bacterial organisms. They work by inhibiting the ability of bacteria to reproduce.

Currently, there is no enrofloxacin product licensed for use in horses. However, the products made for use in small animals and in poultry have been used in horses to good effect, when indicated.

Precautions
Enrofloxacin should not be used in foals. Orally administered enrofloxacin has been shown to cause cartilage damage and joint problems in developing foals, as well as in other immature species.

ENZYMES
Enzymes are proteins that increase the speed of the various chemical reactions that occur in the horse's body (this process is called *catalysis*). Enzymes are needed for many of the body's functions. The most obvious function of enzymes is in the digestive process, where enzymes help break down plant proteins so that the component amino acids can be absorbed (see Amino Acid, p. 37).

Some feed supplements for the horse add digestive enzymes to the usual mix of vitamins, minerals and amino acids. Enzymes such as amylase, lipase, cellulase and pepsin are without question important for the horse's normal digestive function. However, not all digestion in the horse occurs as a result of enzymes.

The problem with the idea of adding enzymes to horse feed is that they are proteins. The horse's body breaks down proteins as a part of the digestive process. The breakdown begins in the horse's stomach, where the proteins are confronted with, among other things, hydrochloric acid. Whether or not supplemental enzymes can pass through the stomach and maintain their effectiveness is questionable.

Horse digestion is quite complex. In addition to the enzymes and stomach acids in the upper part of the horse's digestive tract, horses also use bacteria that live in the posterior part of their digestive system to ferment feed (much like cattle do in the front part of their digestive tracts). The feed that the horse eats is, therefore, actually subjected to two different digestive processes. This digestive process is rather efficient and allows horses to get nutrients from things that people could never digest—like hay, for example.

Enzyme deficiencies have never been demonstrated in the horse. The benefits of adding additional enzymes to the horse's diet are certainly open to question.

EPINEPHRINE (Adrenaline)

Epinephrine, also sometimes called *adrenaline,* is a hormone and a substance that helps transmit nervous impulses. The Latin roots *ad-* (plus) *renes* and the Greek roots *epi-* (plus) *nephros* both literally mean "on/to the kidney," referring to the adrenal gland, which secretes epinephrine. Epinephrine plays a central role in short-term stress reactions; that is, the "flight or fight" responses to threatening, exciting or environmental stimuli such as loud noise or bright light.

In equine medicine, epinephrine is mostly used to treat *anaphylactic allergic reactions.* It is also sometimes included in a dilute solution with lidocaine, a local anesthetic (see Lidocaine, p. 125), where it is included to constrict small blood vessels so as to help decrease bleeding, particularly during wound repair procedures.

EPSOM SALTS (Magnesium Sulfate)

Epsom salts are available as a bulk salt that must be dissolved in water prior to use. Epsom salts have two primary uses in the horse. They are commonly used for soothing and treatment of local infection or inflammation, particularly in the hoof. They are also used by some veterinarians in the treatment of abdominal pain (*colic*), particularly in the treatment of intestinal impactions.

In the treatment of colic, epsom salts serve to draw water into the intestine by a process called *osmosis*. Oral dosing of epsom salts is usually accompanied by intravenous (IV) fluid administration to help increase this osmotic effect. Undiluted epsom salts can damage the intestinal lining. They must be mixed with water prior to administration by a nasogastric tube. However, the true effectiveness of this approach is unknown.

In people, epsom salts are commonly placed in hot water and used as a therapeutic bath. They make the skin feel smoother and softer and are also promoted to help soothe tired or sore muscles (this may also be an effect of the hot water). In horses, probably as a result of human experience, epsom salt "soaks" are commonly recommended for the treatment of conditions of the lower limbs, especially conditions of the horse's foot, such as bruising and abscesses.

What benefit comes from soaking a horse's foot in epsom salts and water is hard to say. There would certainly be no osmotic effect exerted on abscesses through the hoof that would "draw" abscesses to the surface, since the hoof has no circulation and is not freely permeable to water. In the treatment of foot abscesses, some benefit may be obtained by the indirect cleaning of the abscess by the epsom salt solution; solutions of other substances, such as povidone-iodine, should work equally well in this regard (see Povidone-Iodine, p. 158). It is hard to conceive of any negative effect of epsom salt treatment of the horse's foot, however.

Precautions
Therapy for intestinal impactions probably should not go on for more than three days because epsom salts can inflame the intestines. It is also theoretically possible to cause *magnesium intoxication* with repeated doses of epsom salts.

Some horses will not allow their hooves to be soaked in epsom salt solutions. It may not be worth the trouble.

EQUIMAX® (see Ivermectin, Praziquantel)

EQUIPOISE® (see Boldenone Undecylenate, Anabolic Steroid)

EQVALAN® (see Ivermectin)

ERYTHROMYCIN

Erythromycin is an antibiotic that finds occasional use in the horse. It is most commonly supplied in the pill form for oral administration. The drug works by preventing the manufacture of new proteins within bacteria, which causes the bacteria to die.

Erythromycin is most commonly recommended for the treatment of bacterial infection caused by *Rhodococcus equi*. This bacteria causes a particularly nasty pneumonia in foals, characterized by the formation of abscesses in the lungs. For the treatment of *Rhodococcus* infection, erythromycin is commonly used in conjunction with rifampin (see Rifampin, p. 167).

Side Effects

Erythromycin can cause severe diarrhea in horses. This may be due to some effect on the movement of the intestines. At low doses, some surgeons use erythromycin in an effort to stimulate movement of the intestines after abdominal surgery.

ESTRADIOL (see Estrogen)

ESTROGEN

Estrogen is a generic term for any number of steroid hormones that have the ability to cause mares—and females of all mammalian species—to demonstrate estrous ("heat") behavior. Estrogens are formed primarily in the sex organs of both sexes and have various normal functions and therapeutic uses. Estrogens are primarily responsible for the sex characteristics of females and during the reproductive cycle they act on the mare's reproductive tract to help provide an environment that's suitable for the development of the embryonic horse.

In reproductive medicine, estrogens are primarily used in the management of the mare's heat cycle. Combined with progesterone (see

Progesterone, p. 159), estrogens have been used to delay the onset of heat so as to allow for more precise timing of insemination, particularly when mares are bred using shipped semen. They may also be used to time the estrous cycle of mares that are intended to be used as recipients of transferred embryos.

The rare horse with bladder control problems may be able to be treated with estrogen compounds.

Estrogens have also been advocated for the treatment of certain lamenesses, particularly of the hind limb. Some veterinarians suggest that estrogens relax the muscles and ligaments of the pelvis and stifle and may prescribe them for conditions such as upward fixation of the patella, a displacement of the horse's kneecap, or vague and undefined "stifle problems."

ESTRUMATE® (Cloprostenol, see Prostaglandins and the Reproductive Cycle of the Mare)

ETHYL ALCOHOL
Ethyl alcohol has been investigated for the treatment of end-stage hock arthritis in horses. It has been used experimentally to cause fusion of the small hock joints that, when affected with arthritis, can cause chronic hind limb lameness.

Ethyl alcohol, in various preparations, has also been injected alongside nerves and into muscles. As such, it temporarily destroys nerve function by damaging the covering of the nerve (the *myelin sheath*). The use of ethyl alcohol for such purposes—as when used for tail "blocking" in Quarter Horses—is strictly prohibited by breed organizations (see Alcohol, p. 33).

EUCALYPTUS OIL
Eucalyptus oil is the fragrant oil obtained by distilling the leaf of the eucalyptus tree with steam. It is commonly added to a variety of equine products and used in wound preparations, cough remedies, liniments and poultices (see Wound Treatments, p. 196, Liniment, p. 126, and Poultice, p. 157).

Eucalyptus oil has mild properties as an *expectorant* (see below) and inhibits the growth of bacteria. Because it smells good, it is also used as a flavoring agent.

EXPECTORANT

Expectorant agents are used to help encourage removal of secretions or exudate from the respiratory tract of the horse. They are commonly used in the treatment of cough. Expectorants attempt to reduce the thickness of secretions from the lungs and help make easier their removal by normal action of the respiratory tract. Alternatively, they may help increase the production of normal mucus.

Expectorant effects can be caused in a variety of pharmacological ways, including sedative, stimulant (irritant) and acting on the central nervous system. In horses, the majority of the products used for their expectorant action are either *stimulant* or *sedative* in effect. Narcotic expectorants that act on the central nervous system of the horse, such as codeine, are not used in horses.

A number of substances have stimulant expectorant actions. Those commonly used in the horse include ammonium chloride, guaifenesin (glyceryl guaiacolate), sodium iodide, pine oil, potassium iodide and eucalyptus oil (see Ammonium Chloride, p. 39, Pine Oil, p. 153, Potassium Iodide, p. 157, and Eucalyptus Oil, p. 95).

Sedative expectorants that are used in the horse include potassium iodide (it has two effects), acetylcysteine and saline expectorants (see Saline Solution, p. 169). The latter two agents are commonly used in inhalant or vaporizer therapy.

Comments
In human medicine, there is mixed evidence about the effectiveness of commonly used over-the-counter expectorants. It is not known if they are effective in horses.

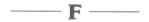

F

FAT

Fat is commonly added to horse diets as an energy supplement. A measure of fat has almost two-and-a-half times as much energy as does the same amount of carbohydrate. Fat is readily consumed by horses and it is an excellent source of additional energy for things such as growth, weight gain and exercise. Fat adds energy to the diet without adding extra bulk. This is an advantage for horses that burn large amounts of calories, such as endurance horses. As much as 20 percent of the horse's dietary calories have been fed as fat with no apparent ill effects.

Fat supplementation has been used successfully as a treatment for horses with metabolic abnormalities of the muscle, such as *polysaccharide storage myopathy (PSSM)*. These horses do not metabolize carbohydrates normally and can benefit from having a substantial portion of their diet made up of fat (usually as corn or vegetable oil). Fat supplementation has also been recommended for horses with *shivers*.

Fat is most commonly added to horse diets in the form of oils, especially corn oil. Soybean oil has also been used in experimental studies. Rice bran is also fed as a fat supplement; it only contains approximately 20 percent fat, much less than the oils, but horses seem to like it.

FATTY ACIDS

Fatty acids are the raw dietary materials for many of the hormones in the horse's body, including prostaglandins (see Prostaglandin, p. 162). Several of them are considered "essential" because the horse's body can't manufacture them. Essential fatty acids have to be—and are—supplied from dietary sources.

Fatty acids are the components of fat. Fat is a dietary essential and a nutritional supplement for the horse (see Fat, p. 96). The exact requirements for fatty acids in the horse have not been established, but all horse feeds appear to provide adequate quantities of fatty acids for normal functioning of the horse's system.

Dietary supplementation with certain types of fatty acids, particularly *omega-3 polyunsaturated fatty acids*, has received a lot of press for possible therapeutic effects in people, including controlling joint inflammation, preventing heart diease, treating cancer and a whole host of other benefits. Unfortunately, none of these effects seem to be repeatable in good clinical trials; indeed, a 2006 review of *long chain* and *shorter chain* omega-3 fats published in the *British Medical Journal* could not find a clear effect on human mortality—that is, patients didn't live any longer if they got lots of omega-3 fats. Nor were beneficial effects seen in artery disease, those prone to heart attacks or cancer. There's certainly no evidence for such an effect in horses, although research is ongoing.

There is one report of a fatty-acid-containing supplement being effective as a preventive treatment for laminitis. Such reports are unconfirmed, and supplements should never be considered a substitute for proper management.

Insufficient amounts of fatty acids have been associated with poor hair coat quality and poor skin health in other species but not in the horse. Regular grooming is always a sure way to help improve the horse's appearance.

FENUGREEK

The fenugreek plant grows wild from the eastern Mediterranean area to China; it is cultivated worldwide as a crop plant. From a medicinal standpoint, the applicable part of the fenugreek plant is the seed.

The uses of fenugreek are legion. Orally, fenugreek may be prescribed to humans for lowering blood glucose in people with diabetes, loss of appetite, dyspepsia, gastritis, constipation, atherosclerosis, high serum cholesterol and triglycerides, for promoting lactation, for kidney ailments, beriberi, hernia, impotence and other male problems, for fever, mouth ulcers, boils, bronchitis, cellulitis, tuberculosis, chronic coughs, chapped lips, baldness and cancer. Applied topically, fenugreek may be recommended as a poultice (see Poultice, p. 157). In foods, fenugreek is included as an ingredient in spice blends. It is also used as a flavoring agent in imitation maple syrup, foods, beverages and tobacco. In manufacturing, fenugreek extracts are used in soaps and cosmetics.

There is no scientific information to suggest that fenugreek is actually helpful for any of its medicinal uses.

Precautions
Ingesting fenugreek has been associated with diarrhea and allergic reactions in people.

Comments
The name fenugreek, or *foenum-graecum*, is from Latin for "Greek hay." The taste and odor of fenugreek resembles maple syrup, and it has been used to mask the taste of medicines. Fenugreek leaves are eaten in India as a vegetable. In the nation of Yemen it is the main condiment and an ingredient added to the national dish called "Saltah."

FERROUS SULFATE
Ferrous sulfate is an iron-containing compound. In man, it is commonly used in the treatment of iron deficiency anemias. Externally, it is used as a mild disinfectant.

Ferrous sulfate is a component of an over-the-counter coolant gel sold for use on the limbs of horses (see Coolant Gel, p. 69). What beneficial effect it might have is unknown.

FISH OIL
Fish oil is an oil produced from a variety of fish species. It is similar in effects to cod liver oil (see Cod Liver Oil, p. 69). It is also a source of *omega-3 fatty acids* (see Fatty Acids, p. 97).

Dietary supplementation of horses with fish oil has been evaluated in a few small studies. Effects on exercising horses, horse immune function and stallion semen quality have been studied, with most studies showing small changes on specific measurements. What significance this has for the whole horse is a debatable question.

5-FLUOROURACIL (5-FU, Efudex®)
Fluorouracil (floor-oh-UR-a-sill), or 5-FU, is a drug that is used in the treatment of cancer in people and horses. It belongs to the family of drugs called *antimetabolites.* 5-FU works by inhibiting the cell's ability to make DNA, which ultimately results in cell death.

In humans, the principal use of the drug is in cancer of the colon and rectum, for which it has been the established form of chemotherapy for decades. In horses, topical 5-FU cream has been used for the treatment of *equine sarcoids.* It has also been used both topically and as an injection for the treatment of *squamous cell carcinomas,* a cancer which can occur on pink-skinned areas of both male and female horses with such color pigmentation.

FLUNIXIN MEGLUMINE (Banamine®)
Flunixin meglumine is another of the nonsteroidal anti-inflammatory agents used in the horse (see Nonsteroidal Anti-Inflammatory Drug, p. 141). It comes as a sterile solution for intramuscular (IM) or intravenous (IV) injection, or in a paste or powder for oral administration. It is recommended for the relief of pain and inflammation associated with disorders of the musculoskeletal system in

the horse. It is also commonly used for the treatment of pain associated with the gastrointestinal system (*colic*).

According to one study, flunixin appears to be approximately four times more potent in its effects than phenylbutazone on a milligram-per-milligram basis. This potency is not any particular advantage, however, as the recommended milligram dose of the drug is one-fourth that of phenylbutazone (see Phenylbutazone, p. 150).

The anti-inflammatory effects of flunixin last from twelve to twenty-four hours after a single injection, long after the drug ceases to be detectable in the system by a blood test. The drug can be detected by urine analysis for up to 48 hours after administration, however.

While flunixin is useful for the treatment of colic pain, its effects are certainly less pronounced than are those of xylazine or detomodine (see Xylazine, p. 198, and Detomodine, p. 78). For relief of severe colic pain, they are certainly the drugs of choice. Some veterinarians report that flunixin "masks" colic pain and makes the decision for surgical intervention more difficult (experimental evidence makes this opinion difficult to understand). Horses referred for surgery should have a record of the treatment given to them prior to referral provided to the surgeon in attendance.

Flunixin is also useful in the treatment of *endotoxic shock*, a condition occasionally seen and associated with severe gastrointestinal infection and inflammation. It is also one of the most potent anti-inflammatory drugs for the relief of inflammation of the eye.

Finally, in reproductive medicine, flunixin is commonly given in management of twin pregnancies, when one twin is "pinched" by rectal palpation in hopes that the other will remain viable. The flunixin is given in an effort to reduce inflammation in the uterus after the "pinch" and to hopefully prevent abortion of the remaining fetus. The effect of flunixin on pregnant mares or fetuses has not been determined; however, management of twins in this fashion has not been associated with any adverse effects on the mare or surviving foal.

Precautions

Horses with known liver or kidney damage should be monitored closely if on flunixin. It should be used carefully in conjunction with *aminoglycoside antibiotics* (see Gentamycin Sulfate, p. 105, and Amikacin Sulfate, p. 37) because it increases the potential for these drugs to have toxic effects on the kidneys. Caution should be used in giving flunixin to weak, anemic, dehydrated or debilitated animals. Animals under 30 days of age have difficulty metabolizing and eliminating flunixin.

There are regulations regarding the use of flunixin for horses involved in shows and competitions.

Side Effects
When used for the conditions intended and in the manner directed, few clinical complications are reported with flunixin. About six times the IV dose in ponies, for five consecutive days, produces signs of toxicosis. As with all drugs of this class, overdose can produce signs of gastrointestinal ulceration. When flunixin is used intramuscularly, there are isolated reports of muscle swelling, soreness and abscessation. Allergic reactions to the drug have also been infrequently reported.

FLUPHENAZINE (Prolixin®)

Fluphenazine is an antipsychotic drug used to treat psychoses in people, such as schizophrenia or bipolar depression. Chemically, it's distantly related to acepromazine; however, it's much more potent (see Acepromazine Maleate, p. 31).

Fluphenazine has gained some popularity in show horse circles as a long-term calming agent. There's no information available as to how well the drug works, nor have standard doses been established in horses.

Precautions
Severe side effects are occasionally reported in horses given fluphenazine, including progressive agitation and unusual repetitive motions. These usually resolve with treatment over a few days.

FLUPROSTENOL (see Prostaglandins and the Reproductive Cycle of the Mare)

FLUTICASONE (FLOVENT®)

Fluticasone (flu-TEA-ca-zone) is an inhaled corticosteroid drug (see Corticosteroid, p. 71), used with inhalers designed for horses in the treatment of airway problems such as *chronic obstructive pulmonary disease (COPD)*. Inhaled steroids are a very effective treatment for inflamed air passages; the inhaled route of administration is considered a topical application of the drug.

Because fluticasone is applied *topically,* the dose of steroids is quite low, compared to what is necessary when steroids are given by other routes of administration for the treatment of airway disease. A lower dose is typically associated with fewer side effects in the administration of any drug.

FOLIC ACID
Folic acid is one of the group of B-vitamins (see Vitamin B, p. 190). It is important for normal red blood cell function in the horse. Folic acid is synthesized by the bacteria living in the horse's intestines in ample quantities to prevent deficiencies, even when a horse's diet itself is deficient in folic acid. Bacterial production of folic acid in the intestines also prevents deficiencies when drugs that inhibit folic acid synthesis, such as *sulfa antibacterial drugs*, are used to treat infection (see Sulfa, p. 178). Signs of toxicities or deficiencies of folic acid have not been reported in the horse.

Studies have been done regarding the effects of folic acid on the horse's *hemoglobin* (the protein in red blood cells that carries oxygen). In one study, exercising horses were found to have lower levels of folic acid than pregnant mares or pastured ponies; stabled horses tended to have lower folic acid levels than did horses in pasture in another study. One horse that had performed poorly at the racetrack reportedly responded positively to supplementation with folic acid. After injection of folic acid, increases in serum folic acid and red blood cell levels were observed in one study, but this effect disappeared in twenty-four hours.

The use of folic acid supplements has been recommended by some in an effort to reduce the risk of folic acid deficiency, but one case report showed that supplementation failed to prevent the development of folic acid deficiency.

Folic acid supplements appear to be poorly absorbed by the horse, and injectable solutions of folic acid are not generally available for use in the horse.

FSH (Follicle Stimulating Hormone)

Follicle stimulating hormone (FSH) may be given to mares for a variety of reproductive purposes. It is used in an effort to stimulate development of egg-containing follicles on the mare's ovary when the mare is not cycling due to seasonal factors, or because she is lactating and not showing signs of estrus ("heat"). It is also used in an attempt to *superovulate* (make more than one egg) mares who are intended to be donors of embryos.

FULVACIN® (see Griseofulvin)

FURACIN® (Fura-Septin®, Furazone®, see Nitrofurazone)

FUROSEMIDE (Salix®)

Furosemide is undoubtedly the most commonly used diuretic agent in horses. It comes as a sterile solution for intravenous (IV) injection.

Although furosemide has other therapeutic applications, it is most commonly used in an attempt to prevent *exercise-induced pulmonary hemorrhage* (*EIPH* or a "bleeder"). This is a condition that is most commonly seen in racehorses, although it has been seen in performance horses of other occupations. Studies have shown that furosemide is only marginally effective at reducing the incidence of exercise-induced pulmonary hemorrhage in horses.

Furosemide is a controversial drug in some circles. In addition to its diuretic effects, some studies have suggested that it may improve racing performance. Effects of furosemide have been noted in the cardiovascular, respiratory and renal systems in the horse. Specific toxicity studies on furosemide have not been performed on horses.

Precautions

Furosemide use is prohibited by racing associations in some states, as well as by the United States Equestrian Federation (USEF).

Side Effects

Excessive use of furosemide can lead to fluid and electrolyte imbalances, particularly potassium deficiencies.

—— **G** ——

GARLIC

Among the innumerable health applications for garlic in people, treatment of hypertension and blood vessel problems seem to be foremost. There is some limited evidence for these effects, but no evidence that garlic is superior to—or even equal to—pharmacologic products intended for such uses. Garlic is also reported to have antibacterial, antiparasitic, antiviral, expectorant and immunostimulant effects, among others. Garlic bulbs around the neck reportedly repel vampires.

Garlic has also been taken orally by people in an effort to reduce tick bites; there is conflicting evidence for the effectiveness of garlic for such purposes. In horses and other animals garlic is most commonly given to try to keep flies and other insects away; there is no evidence that garlic is effective for such purposes.

Side Effects
Garlic has dose-related side effects, which, in people, most commonly include breath and body odor, mouth and gastrointestinal burning or irritation, heartburn, flatulence, nausea, vomiting and diarrhea. Horses eating garlic may also smell of garlic.

Research has shown that, on their own, horses will consume enough garlic to cause a condition known as *Heinz body anemia*, a problem where the blood cells have a characteristic of having certain microscopic features that indicate that they have been injured. The potential for garlic toxicosis exists when horses are chronically fed garlic. Hives have also been reported in one horse fed garlic. The safe dietary dose of garlic in horses is not known.

Comments
There is some concern that garlic preparations marketed to people may not generate an adequate amount of the active ingredient in garlic (*allicin*) to be effective. There is also a lot of variation among garlic products on the human market; equine products have never been tested. Some "odorless" garlic preparations for people may not contain active compounds at all.

Don't worry; there is no evidence that vampires really exist.

GASTROGARD® (see Omeprazole)

GENTAMYCIN SULFATE (Gentocin®)

Gentamycin is one of a group of antibiotics known as *aminoglycosides* (see Amikacin Sulfate, p. 37). These antibiotics kill bacteria by interfering with mechanisms involved in bacterial reproduction. Gentamycin comes as a sterile solution that can be administered by intramuscular (IM) or intravenous (IV) injection. It is also commonly infused into the uterus of mares to treat intrauterine infection and is technically only approved for use in this manner. It has been used to treat urinary, respiratory and reproductive tract infection and also infection of the skin and soft tissues. Gentamycin solutions and ointments are available for treatment of conditions of the horse's eye. Finally, numerous combinations of gentamycin and corticosteroid products are available to treat infection accompanied by inflammation of the eye, ear and skin (see Corticosteroid, p. 71).

Precautions
Gentamycin is generally safe and effective when used as directed. The drug can be used in show horses that are at competitions. It should be used in pregnant mares with caution, due to the potential for kidney impairment and toxicity to the nerves of hearing of the fetus. Because only certain bacteria are killed by gentamycin, it is generally recommended that an attempt be made to isolate the bacteria causing the infection to assure that gentamycin therapy is appropriate.

Side Effects
Aminoglycoside antibiotics (like gentamycin) have two primary side effects. First, they can damage the centers of hearing and balance. Second, they may impair function of the kidneys. Horses that have suspect kidney function, such as those that are dehydrated or very young with immature kidneys, should be monitored closely if this drug is chosen to treat an infection. Care should be taken when gentamycin is used with nonsteroidal anti-inflammatory drugs because of the increased potential for kidney-related side effects.

GENTIAN VIOLET (Blu-Kote®, see Crystal Violet)

GINSENG

Several different plant species are known as ginseng, and some herbal preparations for horses may include various ginseng species in supplements intended for such diffuse (and ill-defined) purposes as calming horses, stimulating the immune system, adapting to environmental stress or promoting general well-being. It has also been claimed to improve athletic performance.

No ginseng species has been shown to improve athletic performance, and information regarding its usefulness for other purposes is limited. No evidence exists that ginseng has relevant effects in horses.

Comments
The various ginseng products are not necessarily interchangeable. That is, effects reported with one species of ginseng may not be seen with another species.

Wild American ginseng is so extensively sought that it has been declared a threatened or endangered species in some states. Some consider the age of the ginseng roots important. In 1976, a 400-year-old root of Manchurian ginseng from the mountains of China reportedly sold for $10,000 per ounce.

The contents of commercial preparations intended for humans labeled as containing Panax ginseng can vary greatly; many actually contain little or no Panax ginseng.

GLUCOSAMINE

One of the most popular supplements on the market today is glucosamine. It is marketed to horse owners primarily for prevention or treatment of joint problems in horses (and their owners). Chemically, glucosamine preparations are one of two salts, *hydrochloride* or *sulfate*, which may or may not have something to do with their purported activity. Glucosamine is often combined with chondroitin sulfate (see Chondroitin Sulfate, p. 65), but it's not known if this combination is any more effective than the individual ingredients used on their own.

Glucosamine is an *amino sugar*, which is part of what makes up the backbone of joint cartilage. It comes from marine exoskeletons, such as crab shells, or it can also be produced synthetically.

Numerous studies have been conducted evaluating glucosamine. The results of those studies are conflicting. Trials sponsored by the glucosamine industry tend to be uniformly positive; trials that are independently funded are generally negative. In the largest trial to date, in 1,583 human patients with osteoarthritis, no overall reduction in knee pain was found between the groups using placebo, glucosamine, chondroitin sulphate or combination therapy.

From a biological standpoint, glucosamine is unlikely to have any significant activity. At the currently recommended doses—even if the substance were completely absorbed, distributed throughout the horse's body, and not metabolized—it is extremely unlikely that useful concentrations could reach the horse's joint. It's also questionable whether a significant amount of glucosamine gets into systemic circulation following oral ingestion. Studies have demonstrated that the oral availability of glucosamine in horses is less than 6 percent; that is, less than 6 percent of any dose is available to be used by the horse. Furthermore, according to the current understanding of the metabolic pathways involved, glucosamine should be metabolized rapidly by the liver or incorporated into glycoproteins. Contrary to what is often stated, glucosamine is not ordinarily available in the circulation as a source of components for building cartilage; cartilage uses glucose for this purpose. That is to say that glucosamine is *not* essential for the biosynthesis of cartilage molecules.

Two studies have looked at the amount of glucosamine in glucosamine preparations for horses. Both have demonstrated tremendous variations in the quality of glucosamine preparations, with many products containing substantially less than label claims. This is a problem for several reasons. First, even if glucosamine were to be effective, if the product didn't contain much glucosamine, it couldn't work. Second, using such products would be a waste of money. Third, the fact that such products exist make reports of their success or failure essentially impossible to interpret. If a product seems to be effective, and there's really not much glucosamine in it, how do you account for that?

It has been suggested that an average-sized mature horse should get approximately 10 grams per day of oral glucosamine if there is a chance for it to be effective; most products recommend far less than that. Questions of effectiveness aside, the combination of inadequate dose and poor quality control makes it essentially impossible for horse owners or their veterinarians to select a "proper" supplement.

Glucosamine does appear to be safe and well-tolerated by horses.

GLYCERIN

Glycerin is a clear, thick, colorless liquid with the consistency of syrup. Glycerin is actually just a type of alcohol (see Alcohol, p. 33). It first came into use in medicine in about 1846.

The valuable uses of glycerin in the pharmaceutical industry are mostly as a solvent and a preservative for drugs. Glycerin is also a moistening agent (*humectant*). It tends to attract water; as such, it is a frequently used emollient for the skin (see Emollient, p. 90). It has a pleasant taste as well. Many liniment, cough and poultice preparations made for the horse contain glycerin for these reasons.
Glycerin is frequently applied to the legs of the horse in so-called "sweat wraps" (see Sweat Wrap, p. 179).

GLYCERYL TRINITRATE (GTN, Nitroglycerine)

Glyceryl trinitrate (GTN) has been used to treat heart pain and heart failure in people for over 130 years. It works by causing dilation of blood vessels.

Because GTN dilates blood vessels, it has been recommended for use in the treatment of horses with laminitis. The hope is that local application of GTN gel will cause dilation of blood vessels to the feet, and possibly help improve the circulation of blood in that area. Unfortunately, at least two studies have shown that increased blood flow to the feet does not occur after such treatment, and its usefulness in this regard is very much questionable.

GnRH (Gondotropin Releasing Hormone, Cystorelin®)

GnRH is an important reproductive hormone that is sometimes used in medicine in an attempt to bring non-cycling mares into estrus ("heat"). Unfortunately, the hormone has a very short half-life in the horse's system; thus, proper use requires either multiple injections or mini-infusion pumps.

GnRH is also used in stallion management. Given prior to breeding, it appears to help problem breeders ejaculate more easily. It has also been used in an effort to cause one or both retained testicles to drop into the scrotum in cryptorchid horses.

In some countries, a GnRH vaccine has been used in an effort to prevent unwanted heat behavior in mares. The effectiveness of the treatment is reportedly quite variable. The vaccine has also been used in an effort to suppress testicular function and male hormone secretion in stallions; however, as with mares, there seems to be a significant amount of individual variation in the responses among stallions, and libido is not totally suppressed.

GRAPE SEED EXTRACT
In human herbal preparations, grape seed extract is usually used for conditions of the circulatory system. Grape products also have antioxidant activity (see Antioxidant, p. 42). Grape leaves are used as a food, particularly in Greek cooking.

In horses, grape seed extract is promoted for such purposes as keeping immune systems healthy and happy and controlling free radicals. There is no evidence that it is effective for such purposes.

Comments
Grape seeds are typically obtained as a by-product of wine manufacturing.

GREEN SOAP
Green soap is a cleansing soap that contains potassium. It is made from a variety of vegetable oils. The green color can come from the oils from which it is made (such as green olive oil). Curiously, the "official" green soap is not green in color. It is very mild and nonirritating. It has limited, if any, antiseptic effect.

Green soap is a component of a popular liniment bath for horses (see Liniment, p. 126).

GRISEOFULVIN (Fulvacin®)
Griseofulvin (gree-zee-o-FULL-vin) is given to the horse for the treatment and control of fungal skin infection. It comes in packets of powder for oral administration.

Griseofulvin is incorporated into the skin layers as the skin cells grow and replace themselves. Thus, the skin becomes toxic to any fungus that is living on it.

Unfortunately, the correct dosage of griseofulvin for horses has never been adequately determined and its effectiveness is unknown. Experience in other species would suggest that for griseofulvin to be effective it should be given for 30 to 60 days. Some practitioners give large weekly doses; most authorities feel that this is inappropriate.

GUAIACOL

Guaiacol (GWHY-a-call) is obtained from creosote. It has some use as an expectorant and a local anesthetic in humans.

In horses, guaiacol is a component of a popular over-the-counter poultice preparation (see Poultice, p. 157). Its usefulness or purpose is unknown in this type of medication.

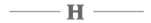

HEMLOCK OIL (see Pine Oil)

"HOMEOPATHIC"

Over 200 years ago, a German physician named Samuel Hahnemann rebelled against the current medical practices of his day. Those practices included bleeding, burning and administering nearly toxic doses of mercury. Hahnemann devised a system of medicine based on the belief that medicinal substances had "vital force" that acted "spiritually" on the causes of disease (which he did not know). Hahnemann took substances that he thought to be medicinal—things like poision ivy, crushed bees or duck liver—and diluted them far past the point where a single molecule of the original substance existed. He shook the substances up between dilutions, banged them against a leather book, and pronounced them to be powerful medications. He called his approach to medicine "homeopathy."

Over the years, and with the advent of modern medicine, homeopathic remedies ultimately declined in popularity. However, with the rise of "alternative" approaches to medicine in the late twentieth century, homeopathic remedies again became more readily available.

As one might be inclined to suspect, since the system is based on the practice of diluting a substance to where it is water (or water placed on a sugar tablet), it has been essentially impossible to show that homeopathic remedies have any relevant therapeutic effect. Indeed, in 2005, in the largest analysis to date of 110 trials of homeopathy, an article published in the prestigious British medical journal *The Lancet* concluded, "... the clinical effects of homoeopathy are placebo effects" (Shang et al. 2005).

Some homeopathic preparations may be given to horses. No homeopathic remedy has been shown to be effective for any condition of horses in sound scientific trials.

Comments
The above information is unlikely to dissuade those who have strong beliefs in the effectiveness of homeopathic preparations.

HOOF DRESSINGS
An amazing variety of preparations are available to apply to horse hooves. Hoof dressings are painted or rubbed onto the hoof in an effort to improve hoof quality and hoof pliability (suppleness). At least one over-the-counter hoof dressing even purports to increase hoof growth.

Hoof tissue is largely comprised of a hard, dead protein known as *keratin*. Since hoof tissue is dead, it has no metabolic function and no ability to maintain itself. Hoof has a very important function, of course, in protecting the bones and sensitive structures of the horse's foot.

Ideally, horse hoof is firm, pliable and not brittle. Unfortunately, many horses are not lucky enough to have "ideal" hooves. Since the horse's hoof is so important, if it is perceived as less than ideal in quality, horse owners commonly try to improve it by using hoof dressings, hoof supplements or both.

Hoof quality is dramatically affected by the horse's environment. Either dry or moist conditions can affect it. Dry conditions tend to dehydrate hoof tissue. Moist conditions can cause hoof to soften or lose surface cells, much like when your hand stays in water for too long and the skin becomes waterlogged.

Hoof dressings are largely composed of the following ingredients: lanolin, various oils, water, stearic acid derivatives, cetyl alcohol, methyl- and propylparaben and petrolatum (petroleum jelly). These agents all act as emollients or as ointment bases (see Emollient,

p. 90). Presumably, just about any oily or emollient substance would have the same effect on horse hoof helping to maintain water content. One study of such preparations concluded that petroleum-based preparations help prevent moisture loss from the hoof better than do lanolin-based preparations.

The addition of substances such as vitamins and protein to various hoof dressings would seem to be of little use. Since hoof tissue is dead anyway, no amount of vitamins or proteins will serve to bring it back to life. Certainly, applying anything to the dead surface tissue of the hoof will not help speed or improve hoof growth.

Mild "blisters" of the coronary band are occasionally recommended to increase the speed of hoof growth (see Blister, p. 52). Evidently, by inflaming the coronary band, it is hoped that hoof growth will be accelerated, presumably by increasing circulation to the coronary band. There is no evidence that this treatment is effective.

HOOF SUPPLEMENTS
In addition to things that are put on the hoof (see Hoof Dressings, above), things are also put in the horse (in the feed) in attempts to improve hoof growth and quality. Substances commonly added to the horse's diet to "help" hoof growth include: biotin, methionine and other amino acids, gelatin and various vitamins and minerals (see Biotin, p. 52, and Amino Acids, p. 37). Experimentally, biotin has been the only feed additive that has shown any effectiveness in improving hoof quality.

HUMAN CHORIONIC GONADOTROPIN (HCG)
Human chorionic gonadotropin is a hormone that is used in reproductive management of the broodmare. It comes as a sterile powder that is mixed with sterile water to provide a solution for intramuscular (IM) or intravenous (IV) administration.

When it is injected into mares, HCG has been demonstrated to reduce the length of the estrous ("heat") cycle by two to four days. Within about 39 hours (on average) after injection of HCG in susceptible mares, the ovaries are stimulated to release an egg (*ovulation*). HCG works best when the follicle on the ovary (the follicle is the structure from which the egg is produced) is of an appropriate size, usually no sooner than day two or three after the beginning of estrus. This effect on ovulation is very useful when trying to decrease the number of inseminations per heat cycle or when trying to time mating and the release of the egg by the mare's ovary.

HCG injections have also been used in an effort to make retained testicles descend into the scrotum of cryptorchid prepubertal colts. HCG challenge tests have also been used for the evaluation of the presence of testicular tissue in male horses that are suspected of being cryptorchids.

Precautions
Human chorionic gonadotropin is a protein obtained from the urine of pregnant women. Because it is a protein, it has the potential to stimulate an immune response in the horse's body. While this is not harmful to the horse, it can cause the drug to be ineffective, since the antibodies produced by the horse can neutralize the effect of the drug. Therefore, it has been suggested that no more than two injections of HCG should be given to any one mare during the same breeding season.

Side Effects
No significant adverse effects in horses after the use of HCG have been reported.

HYALURONAN (Hyaluronic Acid, Sodium Hyaluronate, Hylartin-V®, Equron®, Hyalovet®, Legend®)

Hyaluronan (high-al-ur-ON-an), known for many years as *hyaluronic acid*, is used in the treatment and control of joint inflammation in the horse. It is available as a sterile solution for injection into the joint (intra-articular, or IA injection). A preparation of hyaluronan is also available for intravenous (IV) administration. For the treatment of tendon and ligament injuries, injection both into and beside these structures has been suggested.

Most synthetic hyaluronan is derived from purified rooster combs. It is a naturally occurring substance in the horse's body, and is found in particularly high concentrations in joints, tendon sheaths and the eye. A joint occurs anywhere bone meets bone. Around the joint is non-bone ("soft") tissue that includes the membrane of the joint (the *synovial membrane*). Hyaluronan is thought to act as a lubricant at the boundary between the soft tissue of the joint and the joint cartilage (the covering of the ends of the bones in a joint) as the joint bends and moves.

Theoretically, synthetic forms of hyaluronan have a number of beneficial effects for joints. Most obviously, joint lubrication is immediately improved after IA injection of hyaluronan. However, the product is also rapidly removed from joints, so it does not have a long duration of action.

Hyaluronan is a fairly large molecule. Because of its size, it can apparently impede the movement into the joint of inflammatory compounds by sort of "crowding them out" (this phenomenon is known as *steric hindrance*). Additionally, hyaluronan has a direct anti-inflammatory effect caused by picking up and removing by-products of inflammation (like DMSO is supposed to do) and by an anti-prostaglandin effect (like the nonsteroidal anti-inflammatory drugs). These anti-inflammatory effects may also be advantageous in the treatment of tendon and ligament injuries (see Dimethyl Sulfoxide, p. 84, and Nonsteroidal Anti-Inflammatory Drug, p. 141). Finally, in the laboratory (but not the live horse), hyaluronan has been demonstrated to stimulate the production of more normal joint fluid by inflamed cells from the joint membrane.

There are differences among the various hyaluronan products used in joints (of which there are many), the chief ones being cost and molecular weight. The two differences seem to be directly related to each other—that is, the higher the molecular weight of the product, the more it costs. However, most clinical studies have been unable to demonstrate significant differences between the higher and lower molecular weight compounds.

Injected into the joint, hyaluronan is quite safe and no adverse effects are seen at five times overdose.

The intravenous preparation of hyaluronan was approved for use in the horse in 1993. Unlike the preparations for use in the joint, the hyaluronan in this preparation comes from a microbial source, rather than rooster combs (although this fact is probably not that important). In the clinical study done to test the drug, 46 horses with lameness of the fetlock or knee joints (*metacarpophalangeal* and *carpal* joints, respectively) were treated with intravenous hyaluronan. One, two or three injections were given. Improvement was reported in 90 percent of the cases. Some surgeons prefer to use this form of the drug immediately post-surgery, rather than direct injection into the joint.

However, how, why or if intravenous hyaluronan is consistently effective for treatment of joint inflammation in the horse is not apparent at this time. One study showed no effect of IV hyaluronan in preventing racehorse joint injuries. The fact that hyaluronan is removed from the circulation within a few minutes also makes it hard to understand how the product *could* be effective.

Precautions
After injection of hyaluronan, either in the joint or in the vein, resting the horse may be recommended prior to gradually resuming normal athletic activity.

Side Effects
Injection of hyaluronan into a joint may cause acute inflammation of the joint (known as "joint flare"). Signs of joint flare include heat, swelling and pain of the affected joint. This effect is usually temporary but it must be distinguished from a joint infection, a serious result that is possible following injection of any substance into a joint. Injection of any foreign substance into a joint should be preceded by proper procedures to ensure cleanliness and help prevent infection.

No adverse side effects were reported in the clinical trials of horses receiving the intravenous preparation of hyaluronan.

HYDROGEN PEROXIDE
Hydrogen peroxide is a germicide that many people reach for when they see a wound on their horse. Hydrogen peroxide kills bacteria by releasing tissue oxygen. The release of oxygen is why, when hydrogen peroxide is applied to a wound, the surface of the wound bubbles and foams.

Hydrogen peroxide is actually quite weak in its antibacterial effects. However, the foaming action makes it look very dramatic. The foaming can help get debris out of areas that are not easily reached by scrubbing.

Contrary to popular usage and belief, hydrogen peroxide is generally not recommended for the treatment of fresh wounds, for a variety of reasons that have to do with its damaging effects on the tissue and small blood vessels. Antiseptic solutions such as chlorhexidine and povidone-iodine are probably better choices for the cleansing of fresh wounds (see Chlorhexidine, p. 64, Povidone-Iodine, p. 158, and Wound Treatments, p. 196).

HYDROXYZINE

Hydroxyzine is an antihistamine. It is available in a tablet for oral consumption by the horse.

Hydroxyzine has shown some beneficial effects in the treatment and control of allergic reactions such as *urticaria* (hives) and conditions characterized by rubbing and itching (see Antihistamine, p. 40).

No significant side effects or precautions have been reported with the use of hydroxyzine.

I

ICHTHAMMOL

Ichthammol is a mild skin irritant and local antibacterial agent. It also has emollient (softening or soothing) and demulcent (soothing or alleviating irritation) properties (see Emollient, p. 90). It is a product that has been around for many, many years.

Ichthammol is made from shale, which is hydrocarbon-containing rock. The hydrocarbon base gives it the characteristic "tar-like" odor. The *ichth-* in ichthammol is from the Greek word for "fish"; the first shales used in the production of ichthammol had fossilized impressions of fish in them, hence the name.

Ichthammol is supplied as an ointment for external application to the skin only. lchthammol may also be applied under a bandage. Ichthammol is commonly used as a poultice-type agent (see Poultice, p. 157), under the assumption that it promotes the absorption of swellings by the horse's body. There is no evidence that it actually has this sort of effect.

Some farriers report that icthammol toughens the horse's sole.

IODINE

Iodine is one of the basic elements in nature. It is essential for proper functioning of the *thyroid gland*. Very small amounts are required for normal thyroid function. Normal horse diets supply ample amounts of dietary iodine.

In horses, liquid *tincture of iodine* is used because of its germicidal properties. It comes as a 7 percent solution for application to wounds. Iodine solutions can be quite caustic and irritating, however, and should be applied to wounds only after careful consideration. In addition, because iodine stains so badly, it is not a popular treatment of wounds of the horse.

Iodine is a component of various liniment and hoof preparations, where its particular effects are unknown (see Liniment, p. 126, and Hoof Dressings, p. 111). Iodine also reportedly tends to help dry the hoof and many horse owners use it to toughen a horse's sole. When it is applied to the horse's foot, care must be taken to avoid getting excessive amounts on and around the coronary band. Iodine can irritate and inflame this area.

Iodine is also a component of some over-the-counter medication sold for the treatment of thrush. Again, when used for this purpose, care must be taken so as to avoid chemical irritation of the coronary band.

IODOFORM

Iodoform is an iodine preparation. It was once widely used as a skin ointment to take advantage of the germicidal properties of iodine (see Iodine, above).

Iodoform is a component of an over-the-counter preparation used for the treatment of wounds of the horse (see Wound Treatments, p. 196). It is less caustic than iodine and tends to stain less. It is not widely used by veterinarians.

IPRATROPRIUM BROMIDE (Atrovent®)

Ipratroprium bromide (ip-ra-TRO-pree-um BRO-mide) is a *bronchodilator*, most commonly used for the treatment of *chronic obstructive pulmonary disease (COPD)* in horses. It is typically given via an inhaler designed for the horse. By dilating small air passages in the lungs (*bronchioles*), ipratroprium eases the flow of air in and out of the lungs, helping horses with diseased lungs breathe more easily. Typically, ipratroprium is given along with inhaled corticosteroid agents such as fluticasone or beclomethasone (see Corticosteroid, p. 71, Fluticasone, p. 101, and Beclomethasone, p. 48).

IRAP™ (Interleukin Receptor Antagonist Protein)

IRAP is a serum made from the horse's own blood, intended for use in the treatment of joint disease in the horse. The serum contains anti-inflammatory proteins that block the harmful effects of *inter-leukin-1*, an inflammatory substance that accelerates the destruction of joint cartilage, and is thus important in the progression of osteoarthritis.

The serum is obtained by drawing a 50-milliliter blood sample from the horse being treated using a special syringe containing specifically treated glass beads. The blood mixes with the glass beads during a twenty-four-hour incubation process, and is then spun in a centrifuge to separate the serum from the red blood cells. So-treated, the serum contains high amounts of a protein that blocks the effects of interleukin-1 in the horse's joint.

Once enriched, the serum is divided into three to five treatments of 4 to 5 milliliters each. It is then injected into the horse's affected joint once a week. The serum has also been used for the treatment of tendon and ligament injury in horses, although no studies have been done investigating its use for such purposes.

Because the serum sample is derived from the horse's own blood it carries minimal risk of adverse reaction.

IRON

Iron is an essential element for oxygen transport by the horse's body. The highest levels of iron are found in the body's red blood cells.

Iron supplements are commonly given to horses to act as "blood builders"—that is, in an effort to increase the production of red blood cells by the horse's body. This is a case where more is not necessarily better. It is virtually impossible to create a diet in horses that is deficient in iron. Additional dietary iron does not stimulate the production of red blood cells nor hemoglobin, (the protein in red blood cells that carries oxygen).

Iron-containing tonics and supplements are frequently given to horses that have been diagnosed with *anemia* (a decrease in the number of red blood cells). True anemias occur very rarely in the horse. Horses have a large number of red blood cells in the spleen and are able to double the number of their red blood cells, almost literally at a moment's notice, due to this reserve of splenic blood cells. Accordingly, routine blood tests that seem to indicate a slight reduction in the number of red blood cells probably do not reflect a true anemia, especially in a horse that seems otherwise healthy (eating, performing, etc.) A depression in red blood cell levels can be associated with some chronic disease states, but it is usually an insignificant variation from normal levels. True anemias in the horse must be treated aggressively and do not respond to iron supplementation.

Iron supplementation is of little value in the horse. Neither iron deficiencies nor toxicities seem to be a problem.

ISOPROPYL ALCOHOL (Rubbing Alcohol)

Isopropyl alcohol is a commonly used antiseptic for the skin (see Antiseptic, p. 43). It is used in a number of liniment preparations for the horse and it can be applied directly to the skin. It has no particular therapeutic benefit when "rubbed" on the skin and its effects and uses are the same as those for other alcohols (see Liniment, p. 126, and Alcohol, p. 33).

ISOXSUPRINE HYDROCHLORIDE

Isoxsuprine is a drug that induces dilation of the peripheral blood vessels in humans. Peripheral vessels are the small blood vessels that exist in extremities or in the brain; these vessels typically carry blood under very little pressure. In people, isoxsuprine is used to try to help dilate blood vessels to help relieve the effects of blood insufficiency in the brain and other tissues.

In the horse, isoxsuprine has been very popular for the treatment of *navicular disease*. It was initially prescribed because some veterinarians felt that navicular disease was a result of problems with the circulation to the navicular bone; however, more recent studies have concluded that navicular disease is *not* primarily a circulatory problem. Nevertheless, in two studies horses with navicular disease did appear to benefit after isoxsuprine was prescribed.

Isoxsuprine is also prescribed by some veterinarians for the treatment of *laminitis* in the horse. In laminitis, abnormalities with the circulation to the feet of the horse have been suggested as being responsible for the development of the condition. No studies have been performed to evaluate the effectiveness of isoxsuprine for the treatment of laminitis, however.

In spite of all this, recent work has suggested that isoxsuprine *cannot* be effective in the horse. The drug is poorly available to the horse orally—only about 2.2 percent of orally administered drug is available to the horse, and most of that is removed very quickly by the horse's liver. Nor have any significant pharmacologic effects of oral isoxsuprine been demonstrated in the horse. Accordingly, the use of isoxsuprine for treatment of navicular syndrome or laminitis—or for any condition—is questionable at best.

Precautions
It is generally felt that isoxsuprine should not be used immediately after foaling in the mare nor should it be given during bleeding episodes. This is because, if the drug were effective, one would presumably not want to dilate blood vessels where the danger of bleeding already exists.

Side Effects
Isoxsuprine is largely free of reported side effects. Interestingly, the drug is only considered as "possibly effective" by the US Food and Drug Administration (USFDA) for the treatment of the conditions in humans.

IVERMECTIN (Eqvalan®, Zimectrin®)
Ivermectin is an antiparasitic agent available for use in the horse. It is available in a paste for oral administration or as a liquid for administration by *nasogastric intubation* (stomach tube). In the early 1980s, a product was available for injection into the muscle, but it was withdrawn from the market.

Ivermectin works by paralyzing and killing parasites. The worms are then expelled by the movement of the intestines. Ivermectin is extremely safe and has been tested at a ten times overdose. It has also been tested in pregnant and breeding animals and found to be safe.

One of the advantages of ivermectin is that it kills the vast majority of equine parasites, including those of the skin and bots in the stomach. (It has no effect, however, against tapeworms in the horse.) In addition to adult parasites, regular recommended doses of ivermectin also kill migrating parasite larvae in the bloodstream.

Ivermectin may be combined with praziquantel to assist in removing tapeworms (see Praziquantel, p. 158).

Side Effects
Onchocerca species are parasites that live in the skin of the horse, especially around the neck, the base of the ears and the ventral midline. After treatment with ivermectin, allergic reactions, manifested by swelling and intense itching, have been seen. This is presumably due to the fact that a large number of skin parasites have been killed. While not a serious problem, horses can quickly rub out mane and tail hair from the itching. This is, of course, not desirable for show horses (see Dewormers, p. 80). Ivermectin is the treatment of choice for skin conditions resulting from *Onchocerca* infestations, however.

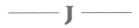

JUNIPER OIL (JUNIPER TAR)
Juniper oil is a volatile oil obtained from the juniper tree. It is a mild irritant (see Counterirritant, p. 74) and also has anti-itch properties that are used in humans to treat such conditions as psoriasis and eczema. Juniper oil is a component of an over-the-counter liniment sold for use in the horse (see Liniment, p. 126).

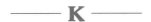

KAOLIN
Kaolin (KAY-o-lin) is actually porcelain clay, made of aluminum silicate. It has been used as a medicinal agent since the time of the ancient Greeks. The name *kaolin* comes from the Chinese word for "high ridge," referring to where the clay was found.

Kaolin is used mostly for its abilities as an adsorbent (it attracts and retains materials on its surface). It is most commonly employed in the treatment of diarrhea of foals, frequently in combination with *pectin*, a fruit extract that is also used to thicken jellies.

Kaolin is a common component of over-the-counter poultice preparations for use on the horse's hooves and legs, presumably in hopes that its adsorbent qualities will be of some use (see Poultice, p. 157).

KAOPECTATE® (see Kaolin)

KAVA KAVA

In people, kava has been used to treat anxiety disorders and stress, among other conditions. Kava has been found to have a variety of pharmacologic effects, including sedative, anti-convulsant, local anesthetic and analgesic activities; however, the exact mechanism for these effects is not known.

Reports linking kava with severe liver damage has prompted regulatory agencies in Europe and Canada to warn consumers of the potential risks associated with this herb and even remove kava-containing products from the market. Based on these and other reports, the US Food and Drug Administration (USFDA) also issued a consumer advisory in March of 2002 regarding the "rare," but potential risk of liver failure associated with kava-containing products.

In 2003, agriculture officials across the United States mounted a nationwide campaign to pull pet food and horse feed that could contain kava. Nevertheless, the product can still be found in some "natural" products intended to calm horses.

Comments
Kava kava was discovered by Captain James Cook during his explorations of the Pacific in the eighteenth century. He named the plant "intoxicating pepper." In the South Pacific, kava is a popular social drink, similar to alcohol in Western societies. Kava is also prepared in a defined ritual manner and used for ceremonial purposes and has been used for thousands of years by Pacific Islanders

KENTUCKY RED (see Carbazachrome Salicylate)

KETAMINE HYDROCHLORIDE (Ketaset®, Vetalar®)

Ketamine is a short-acting intravenous (IV) anesthetic that is used for short-term procedures requiring general anesthesia in the horse, as well as for induction for longer procedures where anesthesia is maintained with anesthetic gas. It was first introduced in 1965 for use in humans. The drug is only approved for animal use in cats and nonhuman primates, but it is commonly used in horses. In humans, ketamine is so safe that it is used for anesthesia of children.

Prior to the use of ketamine, horses are generally given a tranquilizer to promote muscle relaxation. Xylazine is the most commonly used tranquilizing agent given prior to injection of ketamine, but anesthetic combinations of ketamine with detomodine, acepromazine and diazepam have also been reported (see Xylazine, p. 198, Detomodine, p. 78, Acepromazine, p. 31, and Diazepam, p. 82). Horses that have been given ketamine do not appear to be relaxed and "asleep." Although ketamine does not produce a deep anesthetic "sleep," the animals are adequately anesthetized and do not feel the surgical procedures (such as when stallions are castrated).

Precautions
Ketamine should not be used to maintain anesthesia in prolonged surgical procedures. Anesthesia usually lasts about twenty minutes, at best. It should also not be used in animals with liver or kidney problems or in animals with head trauma (it elevates the pressure of the fluid around the brain). As with any anesthetic, recovery should be monitored so that horses recovering do not hurt themselves while struggling to get up.

Side Effects
Adverse effects of ketamine are not reported in the horse. Observations such as muscle tremors, eye movements, sweating and jerking are normal in the anesthetized horse following an injection of ketamine.

KETOPROFEN (Ketofen®)
Ketoprofen is another of the nonsteroidal anti-inflammatory agents available for the horse (see Nonsteroidal Anti-Inflammatory Drug, p. 141). The drug comes as a sterile solution for intravenous (IV) administration. Intramuscular (IM) administration has been reported with no adverse effects; however, intramuscular use is against the manufacturer's recommendations.

Ketoprofen is recommended for the relief of pain and inflammation associated with diseases of the musculoskeletal system. The effects of the drug appear to be maximal at about twelve hours and last for up to twenty-four hours. One 1995 study suggests that ketoprofen is more effective than phenylbutazone at relieving some types of musculoskeletal pain; however, the expense of the drug may limit its widespread use (see Phenylbutazone, p. 150).

Precautions
Ketoprofen appears to be very safe in the horse unless extreme over-doses are given. Precautions similar to those of other nonsteroidal agents would be appropriate (see Aspirin, p. 43, and Nonsteroidal Anti-Inflammatory Drug, p. 141). The effects of ketoprofen on fertility, pregnancy and fetal health have not been studied.

Side Effects
No significant side effects of ketoprofen have been reported during the studies done on this drug.

L

L-THYROXINE (see Thyroid Hormone)

LACTANASE
Lactanase is an over-the-counter supplement that purports to help horses get more energy when the need for energy is greater than the oxygen that is available to produce it (as can happen with intense exercise). The product claims to provide "nutritional factors"—primarily B vitamins and calcium—that are necessary to form *acetyl coenzyme A*, which itself is important in energy generation and metabolism. By doing so, the product claims—among other things— to prevent lactic acid build-up in muscle cells, which is supposed to also help delay fatigue.

There's absolutely no evidence to support the claims made for the supplement, most of which are fanciful under any circumstance. Nor is there any reason to believe that any deficient vitamin "nutritional factors" prevent horses from exercising efficiently.

LACTOBACILLUS (see Bacterial Supplements)

LANOLIN
Lanolin is a purified fat-like substance that comes from sheep wool. Its use was begun by Galen, the famous first-century Roman physician.

Lanolin is used primarily as a base for ointments in the horse that are applied to the skin and the hoof. Lanolin is useful as an emollient (see Emollient, p. 90).

LASIX® (now called Salix®, see Furosemide)

LIDOCAINE HYDROCHLORIDE

Lidocaine is a local anesthetic agent. It is used to infiltrate wounds locally to make them numb when it is necessary to repair them with sutures. Lidocaine is also used for local anesthetic "nerve blocks," used during lameness examinations and other procedures. In addition, it can be employed for anesthesia of the surface of the eye or within a joint, if anesthesia of these areas is desired, and it is occasionally used to help treat arrhythmias of the heart in horses. Finally, intravenous (IV) lidocaine has been used in an effort to stimulate bowel movement in horses that have undergone colic surgery.

Many local anesthetic agents have been developed. Lidocaine is the one that is most commonly used in the horse because it is safe and relatively inexpensive. It comes as a sterile solution for injection in the muscle, under the skin or in the vein.

Lidocaine is also combined with epinephrine in some solutions. Epinephrine, an important hormone in the horse's body, causes blood vessels to constrict when it is injected locally (see Epinephrine, p. 92). Some veterinarians elect to use the combination product in an effort to control bleeding during wound repair.

Precautions

Because lidocaine causes anesthesia of an area, it is possible that damage to anesthetized structures can occur, particularly during a lameness examination. Although it happens very rarely, fractures or other injuries have occurred when injured structures have been anesthetized and the horse begins to use the affected area in a normal fashion. Prior to beginning use of lidocaine (or any local anesthetic), a thorough examination of the horse should be performed to help ensure that serious conditions that could be dramatically worsened by exercise do not exist in a limb that is to be anesthetized.

Lidocaine and most other commonly used local anesthetics in the horse are chemically related to procaine (see Procaine, p. 159). Drugs related to procaine, such as lidocaine, are detected in routine drug tests administered by various competition organizations.

Side Effects

Lidocaine is very safe in the horse. Side effects can be seen in small animals if large amounts of the drug are absorbed, but the size of the horse usually precludes this problem.

LIME

Lime is a chemical (*calcium hydroxide*) that is commonly used in the manufacture of cement. It is also used as a drying agent that is spread on the bottom of wet stalls to help dry them after they are cleaned out.

Lime is the principal component of a popular over-the-counter wound preparation (see Wound Treatments, p. 196). It is used because it has some disinfectant properties (see Disinfectant, p. 88), although what possible benefit could be obtained from applying this caustic chemical to a healing wound escapes understanding.

LINIMENT (Absorbine®, Vetrolin®, Bigeloil®)

Liniments are oily liquid preparations for use on the skin. They generally contain various combinations of alcohol, camphor, green soap, iodine, menthol and many other substances (see Alcohol, p. 33, Camphor, p. 58, Green Soap, p. 109, Iodine, p. 116, and Menthol, p. 129).

As a general rule, liniments produce local skin irritation. When the skin is chemically irritated, surface blood vessels dilate. In people, this brings a feeling of warmth to the area and helps to relieve muscle and joint stiffness and soreness. Whether this same effect is produced in horses is anyone's guess.

Claims that liniments "increase circulation" to areas are not supported by any research. As a practical matter, increased circulation has not been demonstrated as a result of any therapy. Nor has any study been done to show that if circulation could be increased, it would somehow improve or speed up healing.

LINOLEIC ACID (see Fatty Acids)

LINSEED OIL

Linseed oil is obtained from a dried seed, as the name implies. It is a yellow, oily liquid used to formulate various liniments and is also available in an over-the-counter preparation for application to wounds. Linseed oil has no recognized therapeutic properties.

LIPOIC ACID (see Fatty Acids)

LUTALYSE® (Dinoprost, see Prostaglandins and the Reproductive Cycle of the Mare)

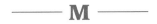

MAGNOLIA BARK

Magnolia bark is an ingredient in Chinese and Japanese medicine that may be used in an effort to decrease anxiety and nervous tension and improve sleep. It may also be fed to horses for the same purposes.

There is no evidence that it is effective for any of its intended uses.

MALATHION

Malathion is a rose and plant pesticide that is also occasionally used for the treatment of external parasites of the horse. It must be diluted prior to application to the horse's skin. It is relatively safe and nontoxic.

Comments

Horses that are intended to be shipped to Hawaii must receive a malathion bath within one week of shipment.

MAP-5®

MAP-5® acts as a replacement for serum and serum products in cell handling and freezing solutions. It reduces the risk of transmitting bacteria and other microorganisms that may contaminate serum products. MAP-5® contains hyaluronan (see Hyaluronan, p. 113). In reproductive medicine, hyaluronan has been used instead of serum or serum products in a number of embryo culture and freezing studies.

Precautions

MAP-5® has been used for intravenous (IV) administration in some horses as a substitute for the FDA-approved intravenous hyaluronan product, presumably because it is less expensive than the approved product. There is no information to suggest that such use is effective, and the manufacturer does not recommend such usage.

MARQUIS® (see Ponazuril)

MECLOFENAMIC ACID (Arquel®)

Meclofenamic acid is a nonsteroidal anti-inflammatory drug that is chemically different from aspirin, phenylbutazone and the like (see Aspirin, p. 43, Phenylbutazone, p. 150, and Nonsteroidal Anti-Inflammatory Drug, p. 141). Like them, however, meclofenamic acid is useful for the relief of pain and inflammation. It is an unusual drug in that it takes a while to take effect. As opposed to the several hours required for the effects of other nonsteroidal anti-inflammatory drugs, meclofenamic acid takes from 36 to 96 hours to begin working.

Meclofenamic acid is used in the treatment of acute or chronic inflammatory conditions of the musculoskeletal system in the horse. It comes as a powder for oral administration. Horses seem to eat it fairly well. The drug stays in the system long enough that once-daily administration should be adequate.

Precautions

In one study, meclofenamic acid appeared to have no bad effects on reproductive function in the horse, nor did it have any adverse effects on developing fetuses. More information would be useful, however, before the drug could be called completely safe for use in these animals.

Signs of intolerance to meclofenamic acid include colic, diarrhea and decreased appetite. If these signs are seen in a horse being given the drug, administration should, of course, be stopped.

Side Effects

At the recommended doses, adverse side effects of meclofenamic acid are rarely reported. Horses have been kept on the drug continuously for up to 42 days and intermittently for up to six months with no bad effects.

When doses of meclofenamic acid are increased above the recommended levels, the number of red blood cells in the circulation is observed to reduce; blood may also appear in the feces. Horses with infestations of bots, a common parasite of the stomach of the horse, should be given meclofenamic acid with caution. Mild colic and a change in the consistency of the manure has been seen in horses that were heavily infested with bots and given meclofenamic acid.

MENTHOL

Menthol is an alcohol obtained from the oils of a variety of mints. It smells like peppermint.

Since the smell is pleasant and recognizable, menthol is used in many preparations sold over-the-counter for horses. It has some effectiveness as an anti-itching agent and as a counterirritant (see Counterirritant, p. 74). Because of its volatile and pleasant smell, menthol is also used for relief of nasal congestion and to make cough drops for humans (see Expectorant, p. 96). Applied topically, menthol is used in a variety of liniments and cough medications for the horse (see Liniment, p. 126).

MEPIVACAINE HYDROCHLORIDE (Carbocaine®)

Mepivacaine is chemically related to lidocaine and is roughly equal to that drug in potency and toxicity (see Lidocaine Hydrochloride, p. 125). It comes as a sterile solution and can be used for local nerve blocks, injection in the spinal canal (*epidural*), injection in joints, as a topical spray and for infiltrating wounds.

A recent study has shown that the onset of joint anesthesia with mepivacaine begins approximately five minutes after injection and lasts for approximately 55 minutes. Mepivacaine apparently does not have a longer-lasting effect than lidocaine, as some people believe.

METHIONINE

Methionine (meh-THIGH-o-neen) is a sulfur-containing amino acid. Amino acids are the building blocks from which proteins are made (see Amino Acid, p. 37). Methionine is found in high concentrations in horse hooves. Accordingly, a variety of hoof supplements have been devised which include methionine, apparently with the belief that if some methionine is needed for normal hoof, additional amounts will make the hoof even better (see Hoof Supplements, p. 112).

Methionine deficiencies have not been demonstrated in the horse. Supplementation with methionine to improve hoof quality has largely been disappointing.

METHOCARBAMOL (Robaxin®)

Although methocarbamol is *not* a muscle relaxant (it is a central nervous system depressant), it is sometimes prescribed for the relief of inflammation and perceived muscle problems in horses. It is used in the treatment of such conditions as muscle injury and *rhabdomyolysis* (*myositis* or "tying up") and for maintaining muscle relaxation in horses afflicted with *tetanus*.

Methocarbamol is available as a sterile solution for intravenous (IV) injection in horses. An oral tablet is also commonly given to horses; however, no studies have been done on horses to determine what, if any, dose of methocarbamol given orally is effective.

Precautions
The effects of methocarbamol on breeding animals have not been determined.

Methocarbamol has the potential to cause sedation in the horse. Because of this effect, the drug has been used in an effort to calm horses, particularly those used for performance. The use of methocarbamol is therefore controlled by organizations that oversee competitions.

Intravenous methocarbamol should not be given to horses with kidney failure because the vehicle in which the drug is carried in solution can be potentially harmful if kidney function is impaired.

Side Effects
Few adverse side effects of methocarbamol are reported. Methocarbamol seems to be quite safe and nontoxic. The drug appears safe at up to eight times overdose. Salivation, weakness and stumbling are reported effects in small animals.

METHYL SALICYLATE (Wintergreen Oil)
Methyl salicylate can be made synthetically or by distilling the leaves of plants that contain this compound. Methyl salicylate is a compound that is useful in the manufacture of various preparations for the horse, such as wound treatments, liniments and poultices (see Wound Treatments, p. 196, Liniment, p. 126, and Poultice, p. 157). It is considered to have little or no therapeutic value on its own, however.

Methyl salicylate is considered a flavoring agent. It smells like wintergreen candy. It has some use as a mild counterirritant (see Counterirritant, p. 74).

METHYLENE BLUE
Methylene blue is a chemical dye that is available as a treatment for superficial wounds in the horse. Other than turning them blue, it has no known effect on wounds (see Wound Treatments, p. 196).

METHYLPARABEN
Methylparaben is a preservative agent with antifungal properties. It is used to help preserve cosmetic preparations that contain fats and oils. It is found in a variety of hoof dressings for horses, which also contain high quantities of various oils (see Hoof Dressings, p. 111). In high concentrations, methylparaben also has an antiseptic effect (see Antiseptic, p. 43).

METHYLPREDNISOLONE ACETATE (Depo-Medrol®)
Methylprednisolone acetate (meh-thil-pred-NI-so-lone ASS-i-tate) is a corticosteroid preparation that is most commonly injected into joints for the treatment of arthritis (see Corticosteroid, p. 71). It comes as a sterile suspension. The drug can also be injected into inflamed areas for reduction of local swelling and inflammation, or for long-term control of allergic reactions where the allergen cannot be eliminated (such as fly allergies).

Methylprednisolone is considered a medium- to long-acting corticosteroid. After injection into joints, drug levels have been found for up to 39 days.

Precautions
When this product is administered into a joint, routine aseptic procedures to prepare the joint should be performed. After joint injection, horses are often rested for several days prior to a gradual return to normal use.

Occasional acute inflammation ("joint flare") is seen after injection of steroids into joints, resulting in heat, pain and swelling in the affected area. This effect usually disappears rapidly but must be distinguished from a joint infection, a much more serious problem.

Side Effects
Steroidal anti-inflammatory drugs such as methyprednisolone have been accused of accelerating joint destruction in horses with pre-existing arthritis. In joints, corticosteroids have been demonstrated

to decrease the metabolism of cartilage cells. However, there is little experimental information regarding the effects of injection of steroidal anti-inflammatory agents into previously damaged or arthritic joints, and concerns about steroids causing extreme joint destruction, which have been expressed in past years, appear to have been overblown. Considerable evidence exists that injection of corticosteroids into normal joints is not harmful to the joint surfaces, although cartilage metabolism may be affected for up to sixteen weeks after injection.

Comments
While there are strong and conflicting opinions, there is currently no strong information available to suggest that one particular steroid is the "best" steroid for joint injection. Nor has the optimum dose of a particular steroid been determined. Research suggests that effective doses of methylprednisolone may be lower than previously prescribed.

METHYLSULFONYLMETHANE (MSM)
Methylsulfonylmethane (meh-thil-sul-fone-ee-il-METH-ane) is a dietary supplement for which there have been many claims made for the treatment of such diverse conditions as osteoarthritis and allergies. MSM is a naturally occurring compound found in some green plants, certain species of algae, fruits, vegetables, grains and both bovine and human adrenal glands, milk and urine.

Methylsulfonylmethane is also an odorless by-product of the chemical breakdown of dimethyl sulfoxide (DMSO) by the body (see Dimethyl Sulfoxide, p. 84). Because of this fact, many people have promoted MSM as a "dietary form" of DMSO. That is, they say that MSM will go throughout the body to help pick up and neutralize anti-inflammatory compounds (DMSO does have some potent anti-inflammatory properties). There is no scientific evidence to support claims that MSM has this effect.

It may be claimed that MSM is a good source of the mineral sulfur (see Sulfur, p. 178). However, this claim is unsupported by published research. One study that involved feeding MSM to guinea pigs found that the sulfur from MSM was absorbed rapidly into the blood stream. However, most of the sulfur appeared in the urine; less than 1 percent was incorporated into serum proteins, which is the primary use of sulfur in the body. Thus, while MSM is naturally present in small amounts in a variety of foods, its contribution to sulfur metabolism is likely to be negligible. Furthermore, sulfur deficiencies are unknown in the horse.

In humans, MSM has been popularized by the book, *The Miracle of MSM: The Natural Solution for Pain* (Jacob 1999). However, there is little published scientific research to support its use, in people or in animals.

METRONIDAZOLE (Flagyl®)

Metronidazole (meh-tro-NIGH-da-zol) is an antimicrobial drug. It is available as a pill for oral administration to the horse.

Metronidazole is primarily used to treat infection caused by bacteria that cannot live in the presence of oxygen (*anaerobic bacteria*). Anaerobic infection is most commonly seen in the horse's chest; the disease is called *pleuropneumonia* or "shipping fever." The drug is usually used along with other antibiotics but is very effective in treating anaerobic infection. It has also been advocated for the treatment of diarrheas of unknown cause in adult horses.

A recent report advocates the use of a paste made from metronidazole for the treatment of *canker,* an infectious condition of the horse's hoof. The paste, which was specially formulated for the study, was very effective in treating this difficult condition.

There are no known precautions or side effects accompanying the use of metronidazole in the horse.

MILK THISTLE

Milk thistle is probably the most commonly used herbal medicine for liver disorders in people, including toxic liver damage caused by chemicals, jaundice, chronic inflammatory liver disease, hepatic cirrhosis and chronic hepatitis. As such, it has also gained some popularity for the treatment of liver problems in horses.

The applicable parts of milk thistle are the seed and above-ground parts. The seed is most commonly used medicinally. The active constituent of the milk thistle seed is called *silymarin.*

Some test tube studies show effects of silymarin and other constituents of milk thistle on various liver measurements. Unfortunately, as is often the case, the effects seen in test tube studies don't seem to extend to whole organisms. Indeed, based on high-quality clinical trials, milk thistle doesn't seem to help when it comes to affecting clinical liver disease. Milk thistle does not seem to significantly influence the course of human patients with alcoholic and/or hepatitis B or C liver diseases, and in patients with chronic liver disease, patients treated with milk thistle had no reduction in mortality, or improvements in liver structure (when the liver was biopsied) or biochemical markers of liver function.

There is no information to suggest that the product is either harmful or effective in horses.

Comments
The broken leaves of the milk thistle plant exude a milky sap. The leaves have distinctive white markings which, according to legend, were the Virgin Mary's milk. Milk thistle is also grown as a vegetable for salads and can be used as a substitute for spinach.

MINERAL
A mineral is an *inorganic* (non-carbon containing) substance that is needed for normal metabolic and biologic activity. Minerals cannot, as is the case with vitamins, be formed in the body. Minerals must be present in the food or be supplemented.

Most feeds normally given to horses are rich sources of minerals, and so mineral supplementation in the horse's diet is usually not needed. However, it is common practice to provide horses with a trace mineral block that also contains salt (*sodium chloride*). This practice is certainly harmless, although if the horse decides to pass the time by eating his mineral block, it can be expensive. Mineral supplementation can also be provided in a variety of over-the-counter-preparations. The toxicity of most minerals is, fortunately, quite low (see also Chelated Minerals, p. 63).

MINERAL OIL
Light mineral oil is commonly given to horses for the treatment of abdominal pain (*colic*). Mineral oil is commonly thought of as an intestinal lubricant, allowing masses blocking the intestine to "slip by" more easily. In fact, the effects of mineral oil are not completely understood. Mineral oil may function by blocking the absorption of water by the intestines (oil and water do not mix). It would thereby indirectly increase the amount of water in the intes-

tines. The increased water would then tend to promote softening of hard masses. Additionally, mineral oil might serve as an irritant to the intestinal wall. In this manner, it would serve to actually promote water excretion by the intestine, which would also tend to soften the consistency of feces.

Many products intended for use on the skin contain mineral oil. Topically, mineral oil is an emollient (see Emollient, p. 90).

Precautions
Mineral oil may be given in the feed. Veterinarians most commonly give it by *nasogastric intubation* (stomach tube). Of course, care must be used when giving mineral oil in this fashion. If the nasogastric tube is placed in the trachea instead of the esophagus and mineral oil is accidentally given into the lung, fatal pneumonia is usually the result.

It is possible for mineral oil to pass around masses in the intestines. Although the appearance of mineral oil around the anus is generally a good sign that the horse's colic is resolving, if clinical signs of colic persist, the horse should be re-examined by a veterinarian.

Mineral oil should probably not be used in combination with DSS (see Dioctyl Sodium Sulfosuccinate, p. 86), a stool softener. Theoretically, the combination of the two substances may allow for the absorption of mineral oil into the bloodstream.

Some veterinarians do not like to use mineral oil in horses that may require surgery to correct their colic. They feel that mineral oil may interfere with surgery or make a clean surgery more difficult. However, most surgeons feel that mineral oil in the intestine does not adversely affect the surgical process or outcome.

Side Effects
Mineral oil is very bland and very safe to use.

MOXIDECTIN (Quest®)
Moxidectin is an antiparasitic agent available as a 2 percent equine oral gel in the United States. It acts by interfering with the transmission of nervous impulses by the parasite. This results in paralysis and elimination of the parasite. Happily, it does not have the same injurious effect on the horse's nervous system.

Moxidectin's primary claim of superiority is based on the assertion that it is better than other deworming products at controlling the mucosal stages of small strongyles (*encysted cyathostomes*), and thereby also useful in reducing the frequency of treatment required for successful strategic equine parasite control. However, several studies suggest that moxidectin is only moderately effective at removing the mucosal stages of small strongyles.

Moxidectin may be combined with praziquantel in order to assist in removing tapeworms (see Praziquantel, p. 158).

Precautions
Compared to other commonly used deworming agents for horses, moxidectin has a rather narrow margin of safety. Overdosing with moxidectin can have serious consequences for the horse. This is a particular problem in foals and other young horses and miniature horses. Moxidectin should also not be used in sick, debilitated or underweight horses. Reported signs of moxidectin toxicosis include coma, difficulty breathing, depression, incoordination, tremors, seizures or weakness. Signs of toxicity are seen within 6 to 22 hours and last for 36 to 168 hours. With treatment, horses that have moxidectin toxicosis can fully recover.

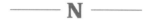

N-ACETYL GLUCOSAMINE
N-acetyl glucosamine is a derivative of the amino sugar glucosamine, which is a constituent of cartilage proteoglycans (see Glucosamine, p. 106). It is derived from marine exoskeletons or produced synthetically. It is intended for the treatment and prevention of osteoarthritis and other joint problems.

N-acetyl glucosamine is not necessarily the same product as glucosamine sulfate and glucosamine hydrochloride. Its use is largely unstudied in any species.

N-BUTYLSCOPOLAMMONIUM BROMIDE (Buscopan®)
Buscopan® (do you want to try to pronounce the generic name? N-bue-til-sco-POL-a-MOAN-ee-um BRO-mide) is an anti-spasmodic drug. In people, the drug is used to relieve colicky abdominal pain that is caused by painful spasms in the muscles of the gastrointesti-

nal or genitourinary tract. In horses, the drug has been approved for use in Europe for more than twenty years. It was approved for use in horses in the United States in 2005.

Buscopan® works by relaxing the muscle that is found in the walls of the stomach, intestines and bile duct (*gastrointestinal tract*) and the reproductive organs and urinary tract (*genitourinary tract*). This type of muscle is called *smooth muscle* or *involuntary muscle*. It normally contracts and relaxes in response to natural body chemicals called *neurotransmitters*, in this case a neurotransmitter called *acetylcholine*. These contractions are not under concious control. If the muscles go into spasm, such as can occur in certain types of colic, this can cause pain.

Buscopan® stops the spasms in the smooth muscle by preventing acetylcholine from acting on the muscle. It does this by blocking the receptors on the muscle cells on which the acetylcholine would normally act. By preventing acetylcholine from acting, Buscopan® reduces the muscle contractions, allowing the muscle to relax and reducing the painful spasms and cramps.

By relaxing intestinal muscles, Buscopan® may also be used to help make it easier to do rectal exams on reluctant horses. Smooth muscle is also found in the iris, or colored portion, of the eye, and administration of Buscopan® can cause the eye to dilate, facilitating a visual examination of the back of the eye.

Side Effects
Buscopan® usually causes a temporary increase in heart rate for about an hour after administration. This is not harmful to the horse.

NAPROXEN

Naproxen is a nonsteroidal anti-inflammatory agent that has been used for the treatment of musculoskeletal disorders in the horse (see Nonsteroidal Anti-Inflammatory Drug, p. 141). It is no longer manufactured specifically for use in the horse, but a generic pill form is available. It was previously available specifically for horses in a sterile solution for intravenous (IV) administration and in a powder for oral administration. Naproxen is from the same class of drugs as aspirin and phenylbutazone but is reportedly superior to either of these drugs in its anti-inflammatory effect (see Aspirin, p. 43, and Phenylbutazone, p. 150).

Naproxen was most commonly used in the treatment of muscle soreness in the horse, such as that seen after intense exertion or associated with *exertional rhabdomyolysis* (*myositis* or "tying up"). Some veterinarians think that it is the drug of choice for back pain.

Precautions and Side Effects
The margin of safety of naproxen is good. Precautions and side effects are similar to those of aspirin or other nonsteroidal anti-inflammatory agents.

NAVIGATOR® (see Nitazoxanide)

NAXCEL® (see Ceftiofur Sodium)

NEATSFOOT OIL
Neatsfoot oil is a light yellow oil that is obtained from the feet and shinbones of cattle. It is primarily used to treat leather.

Neatsfoot oil is also found as a component of various hoof dressings in the horse (see Hoof Dressings, p. 111). The oil presumably has some emollient qualities (see Emollient, p. 90).

NEOMYCIN (Panalog®, Neo-Predef®, Triple Antibiotic Ointment®, Neosporin®, Tresaderm®)
Neomycin is another of the *aminoglycoside group* of antibiotics that include gentamycin and amikacin (see Gentamycin, p. 105, and Amikacin, p. 37). These antibiotics—which come from several different strains of bacteria—kill bacteria by interfering with bacterial cell reproduction.

In horses, neomycin is most commonly found in a variety of preparations used on the skin, in the ear or in the eye. Many products contain neomycin in combination with other antibiotics, antifungal agents or corticosteroid anti-inflammatory drugs (see Corticosteroid, p. 71, and Bacitracin, p. 46).

NETTLES (Stinging Nettle)
Nettle is the common name for any of between 30 to 45 species of flowering plants, distributed mainly in temperate areas. The most prominent member of the genus is the stinging nettle, *Urtica dioica*, native to Europe, northern Africa, Asia and North America. The

plants have large green leaves and most of the species share the property of having stinging "hairs."

Taken orally, stinging nettle root has been used for urinary tract disorders, joint ailments, as a diuretic, for various types of internal bleeding, asthma, cancer and as an astringent (among many others). Stinging nettle is sometimes applied directly to the skin for musculoskeletal aches and pains (where it presumably acts as a counterirritant), for scalp seborrhea and oily hair, and for hair loss and baldness (see Counterirritant, p. 74).

Nettle doesn't seem to be effective for treating urinary tract symptoms associated with prostatic disease in human males, and there's little information to suggest that it's effective for its other uses. As a topical counterirritant, nettle could conceivably cause some short-term pain relief, but how well its application to horses would be tolerated is an open question.

Comments
Stinging nettle leaf has a long history of use. It was used primarily as a diuretic and laxative as early as the times of the Greek physicians Dioscorides and Galen. Nettle stems can be used to make paper. The tops of growing nettles are a popular cooked green in many areas. In manufacturing, stinging nettle extract is used as an ingredient in hair and skin products.

NIACIN (see Vitamin B₃)

NITAZOXANIDE (Navigator®)

Nitazoxanide (nie-ta-ZOX-a-nide) is an *antiprotozoal drug* formulated as an oral paste designed to kill the single-celled protozoan parasite *Sarcocystis neurona*, which causes *equine protozoal myelitis* (*EPM*). The treatment regimen lasts twenty-eight days. The drug is reportedly 70 to 80 percent effective, which is similar to the effectiveness reported with other treatments such as ponazuril or sulfa/pyramethamine (see Ponazuril, p. 156, and Pyrimethamine, p. 165). Nitazoxanide is a member of a class of drugs called *pyruvate:ferredoxin oxidoreductase inhibitors* that block an enzyme essential for energy production in the parasite.

In safety trials, about 25 percent of horse owners reported one or more suspicious adverse reactions to nitazoxanide. The most commonly experienced adverse effects were fever, reduced appetite and lethargy/depression. Some of the horses experienced "stocking up" in the limbs if they were not allowed to exercise. Other, less-reported side effects included worsening of neurologic signs, anorexia, diarrhea, stiffness and colic

Precautions
As with some antibiotics, nitazoxanide can disrupt the normal microbial flora of the gastrointestinal tract and lead to *enterocolitis* and even death. Nitazoxanide is excreted in feces, urine and sweat and can cause pale yellow discoloration of urine and sweat in some cases. This is an indication that the drug is being absorbed. At overdoses, nitazoxanide can cause loose stools, decreased appetite and lethargy. Accurate dose calculations are essential.

Nitazoxanide is not labeled for breeding animals.

NITROFURAZONE (Furacin®, Fura-Septin®, Fura-Zone®, Nitrofur®, NFZ®)

Nitrofurazone is one of the most commonly used antibacterial preparations for the treatment of wounds of the horse (see Wound Treatment, p. 196). It is available in an ointment, a liquid or a powder. Its intended use is for the treatment and control of infection of superficial wounds and abrasions. A related compound, furazolidone, is available in spray that is applied to wounds just like spray paint (e.g., Furox® spray).

Nitrofurazone-based ointments are commonly used in "sweat wraps" (see Sweat Wrap, p. 179). This type of bandage is applied to affected legs in an effort to reduce swelling. The nitrofurazone ointment can be used alone, or is commonly mixed with corticosteroids and/or dimethyl sulfoxide, theoretically to increase the anti-inflammatory effect (see Corticosteroid, p. 71, and Dimethyl Sulfoxide, p. 84). After the ointment is applied, the limb is wrapped in plastic wrap, covered with a bandage and left for at least twenty-four hours. The observed effects of the sweat wrap may only be due to the fact that the ointment occludes the skin.

Precautions
No ointment, spray or liquid, when applied to a wound, should be expected to completely prevent the growth of bacteria. In fact, the

necessity for controlling surface infection in superficial wounds or wounds that are granulating is debatable. However, the presence of blood, plasma or pus on a wound decreases the ability of nitrofurazone to kill bacteria. Some experimental evidence suggests that nitrofurazone delays the rate of wound healing by 24 percent.

Nitrofurazone cannot be used systemically; that is, it cannot be given orally or by injection due to a wide variety of side effects.

Side Effects
Although these drugs are widely used and sold over-the-counter, there is some concern as to their ability to cause cancer in laboratory animals. As there has been long-term and widespread use of the drug with few reported problems, there certainly would appear to be little reason for deep concern over its use. However, the drug has been shown to cause mammary and ovarian tumors in some (non-horse) animals.

NITROGLYCERIN (see Glyceryl Trinitrate)

NONSTEROIDAL ANTI-INFLAMMATORY DRUG (NSAID)
Since the early 1970s when it was discovered how aspirin works, literally hundreds of structurally different compounds collectively referred to as nonsteroidal anti-inflammatory drugs have been synthesized. These drugs are generally anti-inflammatory and *analgesic* (pain-relieving); they also can be used to control fever.

Most nonsteroidal anti-inflammatory drugs commonly used in the horse act in a similar fashion; they block the conversion of a naturally occurring substance called *arachidonic acid* to another group of chemicals called *prostaglandins*. Among their many effects, prostaglandins are important mediators of pain and inflammation in the horse's body (see Prostaglandin, p. 162).

These drugs are among the most frequently prescribed in the horse. Specific compounds that are or have been given to the horse include aspirin, phenylbutazone ("bute"), meclofenamic acid, flunixin meglumine, ketoprofen and naproxen (see Aspirin, p. 43, Phenylbutazone, p. 150, Meclofenamic Acid, p. 128, Flunixin Meglumine, p. 99, Ketoprofen, p. 123, and Naproxen, p. 137).

Side Effects
The side effects of nonsteroidal anti-inflammatory drugs are also

most likely related to their effect on prostaglandins, which are among the most widely occurring chemical compounds in the body. Although rare, side effects are most commonly seen in the gastroin-testinal and renal (kidney) systems of the horse. They also occur more commonly in ponies and foals than in adult, large-breed horses. However, given the widespread use of such drugs, the rela-tive lack of problems is a rather remarkable testimonial to their overall safety when used appropriately.

Importantly, the adverse effects of these drugs are cumulative; that is, using various members of this class of drugs together will increase the potential for adverse effects. Combination therapies of these drugs should be avoided in horses.

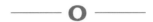

OCTOCOSANOL

Octocosanol (oct-o-COE-san-ol) is an alcohol that is found in some vegetable oils and waxes, most notably in wheat germ oil (see Wheat Germ Oil, p. 194). It has been promoted as *ergogenic* (improving per-formance and enhancing work output) in the horse. It is supposed to increase oxygen transport by the body. How it might do so is unclear.

The consensus of results on studies of octocosanol on humans is that it does not improve endurance. Its purported benefits have cer-tainly never been demonstrated in the horse.

OLEIC ACID (see Fatty Acids)

OMEPRAZOLE (Gastrogard®, Ulcergard®)

Omeprazole (om-IP-pra-zol) is a chemical compound that helps pre-vent the secretion of acid by the horse's stomach. Omeprazole, like other drugs that are collectively known as *proton-pump inhibitors*, blocks the enzyme in the wall of the stomach that produces acid. By blocking the enzyme, the production of acid is decreased, and this allows the stomach to heal.

Horses in race or show training have been known to have prob-lems with gastric ulcers. Omeprazole, which is provided in a paste formulation for horses, has been shown to be effective in assisting in the healing of these ulcers.

For prevention of gastric ulcers, lower doses of omeprazole than are prescribed for treatment appear to be effective.

Omeprazole must be specially formulated so that it is not broken down in the stomach and is absorbed in the intestine. This also means that only brand-name products (no generics) are available at this time.

OREGANO

In people, oregano may be taken for respiratory and gastrointestinal disorders, and many other conditions. Oil of oregano is used orally for intestinal parasites, allergies, arthritis and fatigue; topically, oregano oil is used for acne, spider bites, gum disease, as an insect repellent and for many other conditions. In horses, oregano is included in some herbal products.

There is little reliable information to suggest that oregano is effective for any of its myriad uses.

Comments

Oregano oil has been tested as an insect repellent for *Culicodoides imicola*, a species of insect commonly known as "no-see-ums" or "biting midges." Oregano oil is not as effective as chemical repellants for protecting horses from *C. imicola*.

In foods and beverages, oregano is used as a culinary spice and a food preservative.

OXYQUINOLINE (8-Hydroxyquinoline)

Oxyquinoline (ox-ee-QUIN-a-lin) is a compound that helps control the growth of, but does not kill, bacteria and fungi. It can be used in the treatment of minor burns or scrapes. In horses, oxyquinoline is commonly available in a lanolin and petrolatum base and sold over-the-counter (see Lanolin, p. 124, and Petrolatum, p. 149).

In humans, oxyquinoline is available for the treatment of conditions such as athlete's foot and hemorrhoids.

OXYTOCIN

Oxytocin is a protein that is primarily used in management of broodmares. It is available as a sterile solution that is normally given by intravenous (IV) injection. Oxytocin causes contraction of *smooth muscle* in the horse. Smooth muscle is one of three different muscle types in the horse's body—in the mare, smooth muscle is found primarily in the uterus, the bladder and the gastrointestinal tract.

The mare's body normally produces oxytocin during the first stage of labor. Oxytocin-release begins the process of contraction of the uterus, which ultimately results in the foal being pushed out of the mare's uterus. Oxytocin also stimulates the release of milk in lactating mares. Natural oxytocin-release is stimulated by the foal bumping the mare's udder with his head and mouth.

The major clinical uses of oxytocin are in inducing labor in mares and in assisting removal of retained placentas. In addition, injection of oxytocin is used to help the uterus expel fluid after it has been treated by therapeutic *lavage* (rinsing with antibacterial solutions) and to help the uterus contract after birth or prolapse. Oxytocin has also been used to help relieve horses suffering from obstructions of the esophagus (*choke*).

Precautions
Oxytocin should be used with care if uterine bleeding has been identified. While oxytocin does help constrict uterine blood vessels, the muscle contraction induced by the drug may also cause pulling and tearing that could conceivably increase bleeding in some cases.

Some veterinarians have reported a higher incidence of *fetal dystocias* (where the fetus is delivered in an abnormal position) when labor is induced with oxytocin.

Side Effects
Oxytocin causes contraction of all smooth muscle in the body. Accordingly, signs such as urination, colic and profuse sweating may accompany administration of oxytocin.

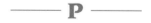

P

P-BLOC® (see Pitcher Plant)

PANACUR® (see Benzimidazole)

PANALOG®
Panalog is a proprietary name for a combination drug product made

by Solvay Pharmaceuticals. It has been made for many years. It is widely used for the treatment of infectious and inflammatory conditions of the horse's skin and to treat conditions of the ears and eyes.

Panalog contains antibacterial, antifungal and anti-inflammatory drugs (see Neomycin, p. 138, Triamcinolone, p. 185, Bacitracin, p. 46, and Polymixin B, p. 154). It is not specifically approved for use in the horse but is commonly used with no reported problems. Generic equivalents of this product are available.

PANTOTHENIC ACID (D-Panthenol)
Pantothenic acid is one of the group of water-soluble B-vitamins. There have been no dietary requirements for pantothenic acid recognized in the horse. Ample amounts of this vitamin are supplied in the normal horse diet and are produced by the intestinal bacteria. The exact function of pantothenic acid in the horse's body is not known.

Sterile solutions of D-panthenol are available for intravenous (IV) injection in the horse. Some veterinarians feel that it stimulates normal movement of the intestines and use the vitamin as a treatment for colic. There is clinical evidence that suggests the vitamin doesn't have any effectiveness in this function.

PAU D'ARCO
Pau d'arco is sold to horse owners as an antiprotozoal agent and an immune system booster, particularly for the treatment of *equine protozoal myelitis (EPM)*.

There is no evidence to suggest that pau d'arco is an effective medication for any condition of any species.

Comments
Pau d'arco wood is extremely hard and almost indestructible. In South America, the Indians used the tree to make bows for hunting. (*Pau d'arco* is the Spanish name for "bow stick.") The anticancer activity of the pau d'arco constituent *lapachol* was extensively researched in the 1960s. The research was abandoned due to the toxicity of lapachol.

PENICILLIN (Agri-Cillin®, Crystacillin®, Aquacillin®)
Penicillin was the first antibiotic, discovered in 1928. It is actually a term for a class of drugs of which there are many members. In com-

mon usage, the term penicillin usually refers to the natural *penicillin G*, which is provided in sterile suspension for intramuscular (IM) injection in horses.

Penicillin G is combined with procaine, a local anesthetic, to help take the sting out of the injection (see Procaine, p. 159). Other types of penicillins do exist for intravenous (IV) injection; however, they are rarely used in the horse outside of hospital settings. Unlike in humans, penicillin is reported to be poorly absorbed orally in the horse and causes diarrhea—hence it is rarely given orally to the horse.

Penicillin G is the antibiotic of choice for the treatment of *Streptococcus* infection in the horse ("strangles"). As such, many misconceptions exist about its use. Penicillin G can be used to prevent the occurrence of strangles abscesses if therapy is instituted early enough in the disease. It has also been recommended that penicillin be given prophylactically to healthy horses in the face of an outbreak of strangles to keep them from getting the disease.

There is no evidence that the use of penicillin G causes or promotes the formation of abscesses inside the horse's body ("bastard strangles"). If a horse does have a strangles abscess forming and an inadequate dose of penicillin is given or is given for an insufficient period, the opening of the abscess to the outside of the body will tend to be delayed, however. Some veterinarians prefer to wait for strangles abscesses that form under the jaw to open and drain prior to instituting penicillin therapy.

Penicillin G is commonly used in association with *aminoglycoside antibiotics* for the treatment of severe infection. This combination increases the number of bacteria that are killed with antibiotic treatment.

Penicillin G is also available in combination with dihydrostreptomycin. This combination is rarely recommended in the horse, however. Bacterial resistance to dihydrostreptomycin occurs rapidly. In addition, the levels of penicillin G in this combination product are two-thirds of those found in procaine penicillin G alone. It has been said the combination combines an ineffective antibiotic with a reduced dose of an effective one. When penicillin therapy is considered, penicillin G alone is generally preferred to the combination product.

Many penicillins have been chemically altered to increase their ability to kill bacteria. An example of such a drug is ampicillin sodium (see Ampicillin Sodium, p. 39).

Benzathine penicillin is sometimes advocated as a longer-acting penicillin—that is, one that needs to be given less frequently than procaine penicillin. A number of products have been made to combine benzethine penicillin with the more commonly used procaine penicillin (Benza-Pen®, Ambi-Pen®, Dura-Pen®, Flo-cillin®, Twin-Pen®, Pen BP-48®). However, studies have shown no advantage to the use of this preparation over penicillin G alone. There appears to be no increased duration of effect with benzathine penicillin and no sound therapeutic reason for using the drug in horses.

Precautions
Care must be taken while giving penicillin G to ensure that it is given intramuscularly. If accidentally given intravenously, penicillin suspensions can knock a horse to the ground or even kill him. As with any injection intended to be given in the muscle, the syringe of penicillin should be *aspirated* (its plunger pulled back) prior to depression. If blood is seen in the syringe, the needle should be withdrawn and the drug given elsewhere.

Injection of penicillin commonly causes muscle soreness or swelling at the site of injection. Horses can get *muscle necrosis* and abscesses secondary to large injections of procaine penicillin G. Thus, most clinicians recommend that no more than 15 milliliters (cc) of penicillin be given at any one injection site. Routinely recommended doses of the drug should be split into multiple injection sites to help avoid this complication.

Penicillin G should not be used in show horses. The procaine that is added to the suspension of penicillin as an anesthetic cannot be differentiated from procaine or lidocaine that might be illegally used to desensitize a horse's lower limb—to keep him from limping, for example (see Procaine, p. 159, and Lidocaine, p. 125). If penicillin G therapy is used at a competition, the horse will test positive for the anesthetic.

Side Effects
Generally, penicillins are quite safe. However, penicillin allergies are among the most commonly reported drug allergies in humans, though they are not commonly seen in horses. Of course, if a horse

has an allergic response to any of the penicillins, any type of penicillin therapy should be avoided in that horse.

Procaine reactions may also occur. Small amounts of procaine absorbed intravenously can cause horses to become extremely agitated. This reaction usually passes within a few minutes.

PENTOXYIFYLLINE (Trental®)

Pentoxifylline (pen-tox-ee-FIE-leen) is used to improve blood flow in human patients with circulation problems to reduce aching, cramping and tiredness in the hands and feet. It works by decreasing the thickness (*viscosity*) of blood. It's thought to work by improving the ability of red blood cells to change their shape (*deformability*). This effect would theoretically allow the cells to go places where they have not easily gone before. This change allows blood to flow more easily, especially in the small blood vessels of the hands and feet.

In horses, pentoxyfylline has been tried for several different uses where circulatory problems are suspected, including *laminitis, navicular syndrome, exercise-induced pulmonary hemorrhage* ("bleeders"), and *endotoxemia* (a serious condition caused by overwhelming bacterial infections). Unfortunately, the drug does not appear to have been very useful in horses in the conditions for which it has been studied. This may be at least partially because in humans, it can take two to four weeks for the drug to have any effect. Also, there seems to be tremendous variability in how individual horses absorb the drug, which makes accurate and effective dosing essentially impossible.

PEPTO-BISMOL® (see Bismuth Compounds)

PERGOLIDE MESYLATE (Permax®)

Pergolide is in a class of medication called *dopamine agonists*. It works by acting in place of dopamine, a natural substance in the brain that is needed to control movement. In horses, pergolide has found widespread use in the treatment of Equine Cushing's Disease (ECD), a disorder of the equine pituitary gland. One of the problems in ECD is a loss of nerve function associated with dopamine, so giving drugs that improve the action of dopamine makes sense.

Unfortunately, the U.S. Food and Drug Administration (USFDA) announced on March 29, 2007, that manufacturers of pergolide

148

drug products, which are used to treat Parkinson's disease in humans, will voluntarily remove these drugs from the market because of the risk of serious damage to patients' heart valves. Thus, in order to continue to use the drug, equine practitioners will have to use compounded sources of the drug, which may themselves become unavailable. Other drugs, with similar function, will hopefully be evaluated as replacements in the near future.

Precautions
Loss of appetite, diarrhea and colic are occasionally seen, but usually only when higher doses of the drug are given.

PERNA CANALICULUS (Synoflex®, Arthroflex®)
Perna canaliculus is a sea mussel, commonly found in New Zealand. It has high levels of *glycosaminoglycans (GAGs)* in it. GAGs are important structural components of the body, especially the joints. According to the manufacturer, feeding perna canaliculus to horses is supposed to increase the level of GAGs in the joint, improving joint function and lubrication (see Polysulfated Glycosaminoglycan, p. 155). New Zealand green-lipped mussel extract was used in human studies for rheumatoid arthritis, but except for one early trial, studies found the mussels ineffective. There is no clinical evidence that feeding high levels of GAGs has any effect on the horse; however, anecdotal reports of the benefits of supplementation with perna canaliculus abound.

There are no reported adverse effects of perna canaliculus preparations. Some horses object to the smell of the supplement, however.

PETROLATUM (Vaseline®)
Petrolatum serves as the base for many of the ointments that are used on the skin of the horse and of humans. Petrolatum also has some effect as an emollient and protectant for the skin (see Emollient, p. 90). It is derived from hydrocarbons obtained from crude oil.

Petrolatum has no known therapeutic properties. It is highly occlusive to the skin; for this reason, it is an effective emollient. Some people believe that applying petrolatum to a healing wound will help the wound grow hair. This idea is simply ridiculous.

PHELLODENDRON AMURENSE
Not to be confused with the common houseplant *philo*dendron,

*phello*dendron is a component of a preparation known as Relora®, a proprietary formulation included in an over-the-counter supplement intended to calm horses (see Relora®, p. 166).

There is no indication from herbal or scientific literature as to why this plant would be included in any preparation intended to calm a horse. In people, it is primarily used to promote weight loss.

PHENOBARBITAL
Phenobarbital, a member of a class of drugs called *barbiturates*, is used in people to control epilepsy (seizures) and as a sedative to relieve anxiety. The drugs, and other members of the barbiturate family, work by depressing the horse's central nervous system.

Phenobarbitol is occasionally used in horses for the same reasons as it is used in people.

PHENOL
Phenol is a synthetic chemical but can also be obtained from coal tar. It is also known as *carbolic acid*.

Phenol has a variety of pharmaceutical uses. It is a caustic agent and can be used to chemically cauterize wounds. It is a disinfectant that was commonly used years ago; other, more potent disinfectants have replaced phenol today. In dilute solutions, phenol is mildly anesthetic and is used to help control itching. Its most important use is probably as a preservative for injectable drugs.

In the horse, phenol is used in some over-the-counter hoof dressings, presumably for its disinfectant properties. Some liquid preparations rubbed on the horse's legs have also contained phenol because it is irritating to the skin (see Hoof Dressings, p. 111 and Blister, p. 52).

PHENYLBUTAZONE (Equiphen®, Butatron®, Phen-Buta-Vet®, Equipalazone®, Pro-Bute®)
Phenylbutazone ("bute") is without question the most commonly administered nonsteroidal anti-inflammatory pain-relieving drug for the horse (see Nonsteroidal Anti-Inflammatory Drug, p. 141). Time and use have demonstrated that phenylbutazone is very effective for the control of pain, inflammation and fever in the horse. It's also one of the least expensive drugs available for the horse. It comes in a one-gram tablet, a paste and as a powder for

oral administration to the horse, as well as a sterile liquid for intravenous (IV) administration only (the drug is extremely irritating if injected into the muscle).

Precautions
The use of phenylbutazone is carefully monitored by the United States Equestrian Federation (USEF). Horses exceeding allowable blood levels may be banned from future competitions. Racing associations in many states do not allow the use of phenylbutazone.

Side Effects
Phenylbutazone has been demonstrated to be a safe and effective pain reliever for the horse at recommended dosages. Its side effects are similar to aspirin and other nonsteroidal anti-inflammatory drugs (see Aspirin, p. 43).

In certain circumstances, caution may be advisable in using phenylbutazone (or any of the related drugs). Two types of adverse side effects have been reported in the horse: *gastrointestinal* and *renal* (kidney). These effects are most commonly reported in foals and ponies; adverse effects are rarely reported in adult large-breed horses. For some reason, phenylbutazone does have something of an unwarranted reputation as being a dangerous drug in horses.

The reported gastrointestinal side effects of phenylbutazone are primarily *ulcers*. Ulcers are erosions of the surface of the mouth, stomach or intestines. This probably occurs as a result of some local effect of irritation from the drug when it is given orally. Ulcers are most commonly seen in foals that are maintained on phenylbutazone (or any other drug of the same class) for various conditions. Ulcers are rarely seen when phenylbutazone is given IV and then only at very high doses.

Kidney side effects are usually associated with decreased water consumption. In horses with kidney disease, illness occurs because of a failure of the kidneys to remove the body's waste products. The use of phenylbutazone should be carefully monitored in horses that are dehydrated, debilitated (and not drinking well) or that have disease of the kidneys. Care should be taken when using phenylbutazone in combination with other drugs that have side effects related to the kidney such as gentamycin or amikacin (see Gentamycin Sulfate, p. 105, and Amikacin, p. 37).

Side effects from the use of phenylbutazone are extremely uncommon at the routinely prescribed doses. Doubling the recommended doses increases the potential for side effects. However, recent research has shown that a commonly prescribed dose, 2 grams twice daily, is not more effective than 2 grams daily, and the lower dose would presumably have a lower incidence of side effects.

Phenylbutazone, as with all drugs, should be used according to your veterinarian's recommendations.

PHOSPHORUS

Phosphorus is a mineral required for normal development of the skeleton of the horse as well as for various metabolic functions. About 8 percent of the horse's phosphorus is contained in the bones and teeth. Its levels in the body are closely associated with calcium levels. The horse's body tries to maintain a relatively constant ratio between the two minerals (see Calcium, p. 57).

A deficiency of phosphorus produces problems with bone growth in young horses and softening of the bones in older ones. These changes are similar to those seen with calcium deficiencies.

An excess of phosphorus causes calcium absorption to be decreased by the horse's intestines. This condition was occasionally seen years ago but reports are rare now. The clinical disease was called "big head" or "bran disease" (it was commonly seen in horses eating a diet consisting almost exclusively of wheat bran around the turn of the twentieth century); the medical term for the disease is *nutritional secondary hyperparathyroidism*.

The dietary requirements for phosphorus are generally supplied in a normal horse's diet. However, some attention must be paid to the "balance" between calcium and phosphorus in the diet, especially in growing foals. Ratios from 1:1 (calcium level:phosphorus level) to 6:1 can be fed with no adverse effects on the growing horse as long as the absolute dietary requirements for both phosphorus and calcium are met.

Alfalfa hay tends to have high levels of calcium relative to phosphorus. Grains and brans tend to have higher phosphorus levels relative to calcium.

PINE OIL (Pine Needle Oil, Mentholated Syrup of Mite Pine)

Pine oil comes from distilling various pine needles with steam. The oil is primarily used in perfume and as a flavoring agent.

In humans, pine oil is also used in the treatment of bronchitis, where it is inhaled. In horses, pine oils are used in formulating some cough and liniment preparations (see Liniment, p. 126). It would seem to have limited use for these purposes.

PINE TAR

Pine tar is obtained by distilling wood of certain species of pine trees. Its use was first reported in the early eighteenth century, when it was said to cure literally every ailment known to man.

Pine tar has mild counterirritant and local antibacterial effects (see Counterirritant, p. 74). It is most commonly applied to the hoof of the horse, particularly under horseshoe pads, in an effort to toughen the hoof or to control the growth of bacteria under the pad.

PIPERAZINE

Piperazine is an antiparasitic agent that has been used since the 1950s. It kills relatively few internal parasites of the horse. Its actions are largely limited to ascarid infections, although it does have some effect on strongyles and pinworms. (Ascarid infections can be problematic in foals and young horses.) Due to the advent of more effective deworming products, piperazine is rarely used by veterinarians, but it is still available for sale to horse owners in pelleted preparations that are fed orally.

Piperazine works by paralyzing or narcotizing the parasites, which are then swept out of the intestines by fecal material and the normal propulsive movements of the bowel.

Precautions
Piperazine should not be used if extremely heavy ascarid infestations are suspected. The drug causes rapid death of the parasites in the intestines and intestinal blockages have occurred. Benzimidazole antiparasitic agents cause a slower, more prolonged death of the parasites and would be preferred in these circumstances.

Side Effects
Piperazine is extremely safe at six to seven times the recommended dose and it can even be used on very young horses.

PITCHER PLANT (Sarapin®, P-Bloc®)
The pitcher plant (*Sarraceniaceae sp.*) is the source of a sterile, watery solution that is promoted as an agent to block pain in horses and other species (including humans). It is most commonly given by injection into muscles or along peripheral nerves.

Little information about pitcher plant preparations is available in veterinary literature. It is most commonly used in injections along the horse's back to relieve back spasms and in injections along the nerves running to the heel of the horse's foot in attempt to temporarily relieve heel soreness. One study, in normal horses, indicated that the product did not cause a difference in reaction to a painful stimulus when it was injected into nerves of the foot.

There are no reports of adverse effects to sarapin.

Precautions
Pitcher plant preparations can reportedly be detected in drug-screening tests.

POLYMIXIN B (Neosporin®, Mycotracin®, Neobacimyx®, Panalog®, Vetropolycin®)
Polymixin B is an antibiotic that has limited use in the horse because it is not well-absorbed from the horse's gastrointestinal (GI) tract. It works by disrupting the structure of bacterial cell membranes. Polymixin B kills relatively few bacteria; however, it is very effective in killing the bacteria that are sensitive to it. Some clinicians find the drug of use for the treatment of infectious diarrhea, usually in hospital settings. Polymixin B is available in various ointments and also can be obtained in pure liquid form.

Polymixin B is the antibiotic of choice for the treatment of infection caused by a bacteria called *Pseudomonas*. These bacterial infections most often occur in the eye or the uterus of the mare.

Polymixin B is frequently combined with bacitracin and neomycin, other antibiotics that increase the number of bacteria killed compared to each antibiotic alone (see Bacitracin, p. 46, and Neomycin,

p. 138). It is also frequently combined with corticosteroid anti-inflammatory agents (see Corticosteroid, p. 71).

Comments
It's called Polymixin "B" because several polymixins have been identified: "A," "B," "C," "D," "E," and, for some reason, "M." Only "B" and "E" have any clinical use.

POLYSULFATED GLYCOSAMINOGLYCAN (PSGAG, Adequan®)

Polysulfated glycosaminoglycan (PSGAG) is chemically similar to substances that occur in normal joint cartilage (*mucopolysaccharides*). Two preparations of PSGAG are available for the horse. Both are sterile solutions. One solution is injected directly into joints and the other is given intramuscularly (IM).

PSGAG inhibits enzymes that are released during joint inflammation. Inflammatory enzymes break down and degrade joint cartilage, which ultimately impairs joint function. Experimentally, when horse knee joints that have been inflamed by injecting a chemical into them are treated with PSGAG, protein levels in the inflamed joints are reduced and the thickness (*viscosity*) of the joint fluid is increased. In the laboratory, but not necessarily in the horse, PSGAG causes the lining cells of the joint membrane (*synovial cells*) to increase production of hyaluronan (see Hyaluronan, p. 113). It may also stimulate the synthesis of *glycosaminoglycans* by cartilage cells.

PSGAG has been evaluated extensively but its actual effects in the horse are still relatively poorly understood. Unfortunately, for all of the good things that can be observed in the laboratory, the clinical benefits of PSGAG are more difficult to measure. PSGAG does appear to be an excellent anti-inflammatory drug when it is injected into joints that have been treated with a chemical to cause inflammation. However, PSGAG has not shown any obvious beneficial effects on healing when it is injected into joints where defects in the cartilage have been surgically created.

The effects of injection of PSGAG into muscle are even less clear. It is likely that PSGAG does reach concentrations in horse joints when it is injected into the muscle. It is possible that it exerts some anti-inflammatory effect and that multiple joints may be affected by a single IM injection. However, it is also likely that the effect on a particular joint will be less than if PSGAG is given directly into that joint. It is unlikely, however, that PSGAG given into the muscle has any significant effect on delaying the development of, or helping in the repair of damaged, arthritic joints. There is no evidence whatsoever to suggest that routine administration of PSGAG to normal horses will prevent the development of joint problems such as osteoarthritis.

PSGAG has been injected in the muscle and injected directly into tendons and ligaments after injury to those structures. Unfortunately, one large study showed no difference between the recovery of horses with tendon injuries treated and those not treated with PSGAG.

Dilute PSGAG solutions have also been used topically to treat eye inflammation in animals.

Side Effects
Injections of PSGAG into horse joints have been associated with inflammatory joint reactions, similar to allergic reactions in the joint. These usually are self-limiting. They must be differentiated from joint infection, which is much more serious. PSGAG injections may also increase the potential for bacteria to cause joint infections, should bacteria be introduced into the joint by the injection process.

The IM use of PSGAG appears to be largely safe.

PONAZURIL (Marquis®)
Ponazuril is an antiprotozoal agent used for the treatment of of the protozoan parasite *Sarcocystis neurona*, the parasite that causes *equine protozoal myeloencephalitis (EPM)* in horses. Ponazuril interferes with normal parasite division. It is provided as a paste for oral administration.

Precautions
In the field studies conducted for approval of ponazuril, eight animals were noted to have unusual daily observations. Two horses exhibited blisters on the nose and mouth at some point in the field study, three animals showed a skin rash or hives for up to eighteen days, one animal had loose stool throughout the treatment period, one had a mild colic episode and one animal had a seizure while on

medication. The association of these reactions to treatment was not established.

POTASSIUM IODIDE
Potassium iodide is a chemical used in a variety of medications and preparations for the horse. Its chief use is as an expectorant that helps liquify thick mucus in respiratory disease (see Expectorant, p. 96). It can also be applied to the skin, where it has mild anti-fungal properties.

An old treatment for *thrush* (an infection of the horse's foot) involves applying potassium iodide to the foot and then pouring on liquid turpentine. The resulting purple smoke is quite dramatic and the treatment does kill bacteria in the foot. This application of potassium iodide can burn the skin of the lower limb, so it should be used carefully, if at all.

POULTICE (Numotizine®, Up-Tite®, Animalintex®)
Poultices are moist substances that are commonly applied to the limbs and hooves of the horse. They are typically made up of clay or other earthen materials mixed with many other substances such as glycerin, kaolin, boric acid, aloe vera and oils of such things as peppermint and wintergreen (see Glycerin, p. 108, Boric Acid, p. 54, Aloe, p. 35, Kaolin, p. 121, and Wintergreen Oil, p. 195).

Poultices are commonly used in an effort to help reduce limb swelling or foot soreness in horses. As the agents dry, it is possible that they tend to dehydrate the surface tissue or absorb surface fluid into them. The actual medical benefits of poultices are unknown. Poultices almost certainly do not "draw out" tissue infection such as abscesses. How such an effect would be possible is difficult to imagine because tissue is not permeable by poultice, which is good, since absorption of clay or other earthen materials into the circulation would presumably be very bad for the horse's health. Also, since no substance can freely move back and forth across body tissue, an osmotic effect on abscesses should not be possible. Poultices should not be able to bring fluid underneath the skin to the surface.

In human medicine, poultices are generally warm, moist mixtures of such things as hot water and linseed meal. These are frequently applied between layers of cloth or muslin. The purpose of a poultice is to keep the treated areas hot and moist; this can certainly feel good in certain cases, as could, say, a nice hot bath. In this manner, poultices increase tissue heat but may cause some local skin irritation. Interestingly, warm applications of poultice are rarely used in the horse. Cold commercially made poultice preparations are those that seem to be most frequently used.

POVIDONE-IODINE (Betadine®, Prodine®, Vetadine®)
Povidone-iodine solutions and soaps are almost certainly the antiseptic agents most frequently used in the horse. Povidone is a dispersing and suspending agent that, when heated with iodine, forms a compound that has about 10 percent of undiluted iodine activity.

Povidone-iodine compound is therefore often referred to as "tamed" iodine. Povidone-iodine has all of the beneficial antiseptic effects of iodine but virtually none of the undesirable qualities, such as tissue irritation and staining.

Povidone-iodine preparations are useful in removing germs from the skin for the treatment of skin diseases, for cleansing prior to surgical and injection procedures and for wound care. It can also be used for disinfection of stalls and equipment. Povidone-iodine is available in solutions, solution-containing soaps and in ointments.

Side Effects
Frequent use of povidone-iodine shampoos is reported to cause drying of the hair coat in horses. They can also be irritating to human skin.

PRAZIQUANTEL (Equimax®, Zimectrin Gold®, ComboCare®)
Praziquantel is a deworming agent developed in laboratories for parasitological research of Bayer AG in Germany in the mid 1970s. How praziquantel works is not exactly known, but there is some evidence that the drug makes it easier for calcium to enter certain parasite cells. This causes contraction of the parasites resulting in paralysis in the contracted state. The dying parasites are then dislodged from the horse by normal bowel activity.

Praziquantel appears to have particular effectiveness against equine tapeworms, a reported cause of colic in horses, and is thus included in certain combination deworming products.

PREDNISONE/PREDNISOLONE

Prednisone and prednisolone are short-acting corticosteroids (see Corticosteroid, p. 71). The drugs are available in pills for oral administration to the horse and are effective when used as directed. A liquid preparation of prednisone is available in drops to control inflammation of the eye.

Clinical research suggests that if one of the drugs is to be used orally in the horse, prednisolone is the better choice. It appears to be better absorbed.

PROCAINE

Procaine is an anesthetic agent chemically related to lidocaine (see Lidocaine, p. 125). It is added to penicillin G preparations in order to take the sting out of the large volume of penicillin that is deposited into the muscle with routine injection (see Penicillin, p. 145).

Precautions

Caution must be used when administering procaine penicillin to horses. The drug itself can be detected on tests administered during competition. If procaine is inadvertently given intravenously, it causes a brief period of extreme excitement for the horse (and for the handler, as well).

PROGESTERONE

Progesterone (a naturally occurring hormone) or one of its synthetic equivalents (as a group called *progestins*) are most commonly given to mares. These drugs have many applications for controlling the reproductive cycle of the mare. Uses include: (1) regulation of *estrus* ("heat") in mares undergoing transition from their inactive to active breeding periods; (2) synchronization of estrus in cycling mares; (3) delaying estrus and ovulation in mares after they have foaled; (4) long-term suppression of the signs of estrus; and (5) maintenance of pregnancy in mares that tend to lose their fetuses early in term.

It should be noted that although it is commonly done, there is essentially no clinical data to indicate that giving supplemental progesterone is effective in maintaining pregnancy in problem mares that tend to abort their fetuses early in term. Otherwise stated, there seems to be no reason to give supplemental progesterone to most pregnant mares. In normal mares that are in foal, the placenta takes over production of progesterone from the ovaries at about day 100 to 120 of pregnancy. If, for some reason, supplementation of progesterone is desired, there is no certainly no reason to continue it past this time.

Progesterone has also been given to stallions in an effort to keep them calm. Why the drug might have such an effect is unknown. It is possible that the long-term use of progesterone in such a fashion in stallions could alter their fertility, at least temporarily.

PROGESTERONE "IMPLANTS"
In mares that show and race, suppression of the signs of *estrus* ("heat") is frequently requested. Daily administration of altrenogest appears to be effective in suppressing estrus for long periods and does not affect subsequent fertility (see Altrenogest, p. 35). Intermittent intramuscular (IM) injection of progesterone in an oil base may also be used for estrus supression. However, in an effort to avoid frequent drug administration, dosing with longer-acting synthetic forms of progesterone (*progestins*) has been attempted.

"Implants" of synthetic progesterone are one method that is advocated by some veterinarians. These are reported to provide a slow, continuous release of progestin from a pellet implanted under the skin of the mare.

It should be noted that there are no implants made from progestins that have been designed or approved for use in horses. Among the implants that are used are norgestomet (Synchro-mate B), a growth-promoter used in feedlot cattle. A number of studies have found norgestomet to be ineffective in suppressing estrus or estrous behavior in the mare, even when given in daily doses. Other progestin-containing cattle implants are also used in horses. Their effectiveness and safety in horses have been evaluated in several studies and even very large doses—up to 80 pellets—have been shown to be ineffective at controlling estrous behavior.

PROLIXIN® (see Fluphenazine)

PROMAZINE HYDROCHLORIDE
Promazine hydrochloride is a tranquilizing agent from the same class of drugs as acepromazine (see Acepromazine Maleate, p. 31).

It is available in granules for oral administration or as a liquid for intravenous (IV) administration for the horse. It is indicated for a variety of procedures in which a calmer horse is desired, such as shoeing, dental care or handling mares during breeding.

Promazine seems to be somewhat inconsistent in its effects and so is not commonly used. Some horses show little if any tranquilization after dosage with promazine. The manufacturer of the IV product suggests that a short period of quiet for the horse prior to administration of the drug may encourage a more favorable response.

Precautions
Routine precautions should be followed in working around a horse that is tranquilized. Horses under tranquilization can still react quickly to external stimuli.

Promazine hydrochloride should be used with care in horses showing signs of illness or shock. Promazine should not be used in conjuction with *organophosphate compounds* because it increases their toxicity. If used with procaine, promazine increases procaine's activity (see Procaine, p. 159).

The use of promazine is strictly prohibited in horses showing in competitions.

Side Effects
As with acepromazine, paralysis of the muscles that retract the penis has been associated with promazine hydrochloride. The cause of this side effect is not known, but it is, fortunately, quite rare.

PROPYLENE GLYCOL
Propylene glycol is a solvent and preservative used to mix various drugs and over-the-counter preparations. It is also used in the manufacture of ointment bases.

Propylene glycol has no known therapeutic activity. Many drugs are mixed with propylene glycol in the manufacture of pharmacologic products.

PROPYLPARABEN
Propylparaben is a preservative agent with antifungal properties. It is used to help preserve cosmetic preparations that contain fats and oils.

Propylparaben is used as a preservative in a variety of hoof dressings for horses. Hoof dressings contain high quantities of various oils (see Hoof Dressings, p. 111).

PROSTAGLANDIN

Prostaglandins are a group of compounds with a remarkable spectrum of biological activity. Their biological effects are believed to cover almost every activity of the body. Altering prostaglandin synthesis is the method by which the most commonly used nonsteroidal anti-inflammatory drugs work (see Nonsteroidal Anti-Inflammatory Drug, p. 141). Synthetic derivatives of prostaglandin are also commonly used in management of the reproductive cycle of the mare (see Prostaglandins and the Reproductive Cycle of the Mare, below).

PROSTAGLANDINS AND THE REPRODUCTIVE CYCLE OF THE MARE (Lutalyse®, Equimate®)

Prostaglandins are widely used for control of the mare's reproductive cycle. Synthetic forms of the hormone are used to break down (lyse) a structure on the mare's ovary known as the *corpus luteum* (see below). These drugs are provided as sterile solutions that are most commonly given intramuscularly (IM) in the mare.

During the mare's *estrous* ("heat") cycle, her ovary produces the egg from a structure called a *follicle*. After the follicle releases the egg, the follicle transforms into a hormone-producing structure called the corpus luteum. The corpus luteum is responsible for the production of progesterone, the hormone that keeps mares out of heat. Progesterone is also the hormone that maintains pregnancy (see Progesterone, p. 159).

Prostaglandin is normally released by the mare's uterus when it is time for her to come back into heat. Prostaglandin causes the corpus luteum to break down. Consequently, progesterone production decreases and the mare will again demonstrate signs of heat.

Giving prostaglandins to the mare mimics the natural process. However, for injectable prostaglandins to be effective, the corpus luteum must be mature. Therefore, the drug will not work properly until at least four or five days after the last day of the mare's heat cycle.

The uses of injectable prostaglandin, therefore, all depend on its ability to break down the corpus luteum. Among these uses are to: (1) end situations where the corpus luteum persists; (2) shorten the interval between heat cycles and allow for earlier rebreeding; (3) try to control the time of ovulation; (4) help treat uterine infection by inducing heat; and (5) abort the fetus during pregnancy. Certain synthetic prostaglandins (fenprostalene) have been used for elective birth inductions.

Precautions
Prostaglandins can be absorbed through human skin and could cause abortion or bronchial spasms in people. Pregnant women and asthmatics should handle the drug carefully. If it gets on the skin, it should be washed off immediately with soap and water.

Prostaglandins should theoretically not be used at the same time as nonsteroidal anti-inflammatory drugs (see Nonsteroidal Anti-Inflammatory Drugs, p. 141). Nonsteroidal anti-inflammatory drugs block the effects of prostaglandins. They should also not be given to horses suffering from gastrointestinal or respiratory problems.

Side Effects
After horses have been given prostaglandin, sweating, mild diarrhea and colic signs have been observed. These signs are usually transient and disappear within an hour. Clinical experience suggests that these signs may be seen more frequently with dinoprost than with fluprostenol or other synthetic prostaglandins, although the effects seem to be dose-dependent. Low-dose prostaglandin use on consecutive days in horses has been studied, and seems to be as effective, with fewer side effects.

PROTEIN
Proteins are the basic building blocks from which tissue is made. Proteins also make up some of the hormones and all of the enzymes of the horse's body. After the fat and water are removed, 80 percent of the horse's structure is protein. Protein is constantly being used by the horse. Even though the horse's body reuses some of its own protein, a steady supply must be available in the diet to replace some of what is lost or used up.

Growing horses are more sensitive to protein needs than adult horses. If protein is restricted in a foal's diet, growth is restricted as well. In adult horses, inadequate protein can cause decreased appetite, loss of body tissue and poor hoof growth and hair coat.

Excessive protein intake by horses appears to cause no obvious harm. However, there are studies that suggest that excessive protein intake may be associated with decreased performance. Exercising horses do not require supplemental protein.

Extra protein does not make a horse stronger. Protein is needed for growth of tissue, but extra protein does not cause extra strength or muscle growth. Extra protein is merely burned as fuel or converted to fat. Digesting protein requires the horse's body to work hard, and giving a horse excessive amounts is just an expensive and inefficient way to give him extra calories.

Most horse diets supply more than ample amounts of protein. Additional protein may be needed by horses for growth and lactation if these horses are fed some poor quality grasses or hays. However, alfalfa-based rations generally supply plenty of protein for horses of all ages and metabolic requirements.

PSYLLIUM (Psyllium Hydrophyllic Mucilloid, Sand-Lax®, Equi-Lax®, Metamucil®)

Psyllium is made from the outer portion of psyllium seeds. Psyllium attracts large amounts of water to it and therefore has some effect as a stool softener.

In horses, psyllium is commonly used in an effort to prevent or remove accumulations of sand from the intestine. Horses can inadvertently eat sand when they pull hay or grass from areas of sandy soil. It has also been recommended as a treatment for some types of *impaction colic* (constipation). However, some research suggests that giving psyllium is no more effective at removing sand than preventing the horse from having further access to sand, whereby the horse will remove the sand on his own. Psyllium supplementation is no substitute for good management—horses may still accumulate considerable amounts of sand when fed psyllium.

Precautions
It is recommended by some veterinarians that horses not be fed psyllium for more than three consecutive weeks. Feeding psyllium for longer periods than this is not harmful, but if psyllium is provided to the horse constantly, the horse's intestinal tract may begin to digest it and thus render it ineffective. Dosing schedules, such as daily for one week each month, are not based on experimental data.

Side Effects
There are anecdotal reports of excessive gas in some horses receiving psyllium.

PYRANTEL (Pamoate, Tartrate, Strongid®)
Pyrantel is an antiparasitic agent commonly used in the horse. It comes in a paste for oral administration, a liquid for administration via nasogastric intubation (stomach tube) and a pelleted formulation that is given daily in the feed. Pyrantel causes paralysis of intestinal parasites. The parasites are then removed from the body by normal intestinal movements.

Pyrantel is effective for control of the majority of equine intestinal parasites, with the exception of bots. Pyrantel has also demonstrated effectiveness against the equine tapeworm; the dose must be doubled to achieve this effect.

Side Effects
Pyrantel is considered safe for all horses at up to twenty times overdose.

PYRILAMINE MALEATE
Pyrilamine maleate (pie-RILL-a-mean MAL-ee-ate) is an antihistamine for use in the horse. It comes as a sterile solution and is given by intramuscular (IM) or intravenous (IV) injection (see Antihistamine, p. 40).

PYRIMETHAMINE (Daraprim®)
Pyrimethamine (peer-a-METH-a-mean) is used for the treatment of *equine protozoal myeloencephalitis (EPM)*, a protozoal infection of the spinal cord of the horse. For the treatment of this condition, pyrimethamine is used along with a sulfa-trimethoprim combination antibacterial drug (see Sulfamethoxazole-Trimethoprim, p. 178). Treatment for EPM must frequently be continued for several months. Pyrimethamine comes as a tablet for oral administration to the horse. The two products, sulfa-trimethoprim and pyrimethamine, may also be mixed together by licensed compounding pharmacies into an oral liquid or paste.

Side Effects
No adverse side effects of pyrimethamine have been reported in the horse.

165

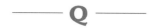

QUERCETIN (Dihydrate)

Quercetin occurs abundantly in red wine, tea, onions, green tea, apples, berries and certain vegetables, as well as in some herbs. It has demonstrated a number of interesting pharmacologic properties in test tube studies, among them antioxidant and anti-inflammatory effects (see Antioxidant, p. 42).

Unfortunately, research in humans suggests that quercetin taken orally doesn't reach the serum concentrations at which the test tube activity has been seen. What, if any, dose is effective in horses is unknown.

For horses, quercetin is a component of a product intended to help with skin and allergic problems. There is no evidence that it is effective for such purposes, and quercetin is not normally prescribed for skin or allergy problems in people.

QUEST® (see Moxidectin)

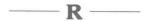

RANITIDINE (ZANTAC®)

Ranitidine is an antihistamine that is most commonly used for the treatment of stomach ulcers in the horse. Its effects are similar to those of cimetidine (see Cimetidine, p. 66). It is available in pill form for oral administration, and it is normally dosed three times daily.

Comments

One study suggests that ranitidine is not as effective as omeprazole at treating gastric ulcers. However, it remains popular because it is currently significantly less expensive than omeprazole (see Omeprazole, p. 142).

REGU-MATE® (see Altrenogest)

RELORA®

Relora is a proprietary herbal preparation that may be given to help calm horses. It normally contains *Magnolia officinalis* bark extract, *Phellodendron amurense* bark extract and vitamin C (see Magnolia Bark, p. 127, Phellodendron Amurense, p. 149, and Vitamin C, p. 193). There is no evidence that it has any effect in horses.

RESERPINE (Serpacil®)

Reserpine is an antipsychotic and antihypertensive drug that irreversibly binds to substances that transmit nerve messages (*neurotransmitters*) in the central nervous system. In the 1950s it was found that reserpine acted as an antidepressant. Reserpine also has other actions, particularly on the gastrointestinal tract.

In some countries reserpine is still available as part of combination drugs for the treatment of hypertension in people, although it is considered a "second choice" drug. The use of reserpine as antipsychotic drug in people has been nearly completely abandoned. Reserpine may be used as a "long-term" sedative for horses. That is, the drug may be given in an effort to keep them calm for a period of several days or weeks. The drug can be detected by routine tests administered during competitions.

Side Effects

In horses, diarrhea is a commonly reported side effect after reserpine administration.

RIBOFLAVIN (see Vitamin B₂)

RIFAMPIN (Rifadin®, Rimactin®)

Rifampin is an antibiotic used most commonly in the treatment of pneumonias in foals caused by the bacterium *Rhodococcus equi*. It is available as a pill for oral administration. In people, it is commonly used in the treatment of tuberculosis, most commonly in association with other drugs.

Rifampin is almost always given in combination with erythromycin, or a related antibiotic, azithromycin. The two drugs given together increase the effectiveness of what is seen when each drug is given alone (see Erythromycin, p. 94, and Azithromycin, p. 46).

Precautions

Bacterial resistance to rifampin alone occurs rapidly. That's why it is almost always given in combination with other drugs.

Side Effects
Softening of the stool can be seen in foals treated with rifampin. While this usually does not mean that treatment should be stopped, foals with soft stools as a result of this treatment should be monitored closely. Sometimes severe diarrhea develops, in which case the drug must be discontinued.

Rifampin can also cause reddish discoloration of the foal's urine.

ROBAXIN® (see Methocarbamol)

ROMIFIDINE HYDROCHLORIDE (Sedivet®)
Romifidine is the newest sedative agent on the market for horses. It is used to temporarily decrease pain, facilitate handling, examination, treatment and as a pre-medication agent prior to general anaesthesia. It reportedly features less *ataxia* (unsteadiness) and incoordination than do agents of the same class of drugs, such as xylazine and detomodine (see Xylazine, p. 198, and Detomodine, p. 78). It has a duration of action of 40 to 80 minutes.

Precautions
Horses under the sedation of romifidine may demonstrate increased skin sensitivity of the hind limbs. Some horses, although apparently sedated, may still respond to external stimuli (that is, they may still kick).

After the administration of romifidine, a short-term change in the conductivity of the cardiac (heart) muscle may occur (a *partial atrioventricular block*). After treatment, occasional sweating and increased urination may be seen as well as ataxia, *hypertension* followed by *hypotension* and *bradycardia* (slow heart rate). These conditions, if present, should be monitored.

ROMPUN® (see Xylazine)

ROSE HIPS (Rosehips)
Rose hips is the ripe, dried receptacle (hip), with or without fruit (seed) of various *Rosa* species. People use rose hips as a source of vitamin C (see Vitamin C, p. 193) and many herbal products contain it.

There is little obvious reason to feed rose hips to a horse. Horses cannot suffer from vitamin C deficiency, because they are able to produce their own (unlike humans). Excess vitamin C is secreted in the urine. There is no condition of the horse known to benefit from vitamin C supplementation.

Comments
Fresh rose hips contain a high concentration of vitamin C; however, much of the vitamin C is destroyed during drying and processing and declines rapidly with storage.

ROSEMARY OIL
Rosemary oil is distilled from rosemary flowers. It is a component of a popular liniment/bathing agent for the horse (see Liniment, p. 126). It is also used as a flavoring agent and perfume.

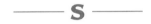

SALICYLIC ACID
Salicylic acid is chemically related to aspirin (see Aspirin, p. 43). However, it cannot be used internally because it is very irritating to the intestinal tract. Rather, it is applied to the skin, where it has a slight antiseptic action. Salicylic acid also tends to loosen and break down the surface layers of the skin (*exfoliate*); for that reason it is often used in the treatment of warts and corns in man, or in soaps or creams to reduce acne and increase exfoliation of the skin.

In horses, salicylic acid is a component of various liniment and poultice preparations that are sold over-the-counter (see Liniment, p. 126, and Poultice, p. 157).

SALINE SOLUTION
Saline solution is a solution of *sodium chloride*—the chemical that is the primary component of table salt—in water. It is generally mixed so that it has the same concentration of salts (*tonicity*) as is present in body fluids. It is the primary component of most over-the-counter preparations for use in the eye. Concentrated saline ointments are available for use in helping reduce swelling of the cornea of the eye; these are available by prescription only.

Saline solution is mostly used in equine veterinary medicine to mix and dilute injectable drugs. Undiluted, it can be given intravenously (IV); it is the fluid of choice for the treatment of foals with ruptured bladders. For treatment of other conditions requiring intravenous fluids, other solutions that are less acidic than saline solution are more commonly used.

SALIX® (see Furosemide)

SAMe (S-Adenosylmethionine)

S-adenosylmethionine (SAMe) is a naturally occurring compound found in all living cells. Commercially, it is produced in yeast-cell cultures.

SAMe plays an essential role in more than 100 biochemical reactions. As such, it has found popularity in an amazing array of conditions in people. Given mostly orally (an intravenous—IV— form is available), SAMe has been suggested as an option for treating depression, anxiety, heart disease, osteoarthritis, bursitis, tendonitis, chronic lower back pain, dementia, Alzheimer's disease, slowing the aging process, chronic fatigue syndrome, Parkinson's disease, some liver diseases, headaches and many other conditions. SAMe has been available by prescription in Europe since 1975, where it is used to treat depression in humans. The mechanism for any antidepressant effect is unknown.

Interestingly, the potential usefulness of SAMe for treating osteoarthritis was discovered when patients in clinical trials of SAMe for depression noted improvement in their osteoarthritis symptoms. SAMe donates a chemical (*methyl*) group that is important to reactions that aid in the production of cartilage *proteoglycans*. A number of studies have found SAMe to be more effective than a placebo in improving pain and stiffness related to osteoarthritis in people. However, from the standpoint of quality, many of these studies were poorly conducted (nonrandomized, uncontrolled, unblinded and some were flawed statistically). No studies documenting disease arrest or reversal are found in the scientific literature. There is, however, some evidence in people that SAMe may be as effective as using nonsteroidal anti-inflammatory drugs, with a lower incidence of side effects.

Some clinical trials have concluded that SAMe can normalize liver enzymes and decrease symptoms associated with various forms of chronic liver disease in people. However, most of those trials have been on small numbers of human patients and did not cover a long enough time period to know if such changes are significant or long-lasting.

Side Effects
There are no standard dosages established for horses. Side effects in people include occasional gastrointestinal disturbances, mainly flatulence, nausea and diarrhea.

Comments
Persons interested in using SAMe in horses may find that it has a prohibitively high cost.

SARAPIN® (see Pitcher Plant)

SASSAFRAS OIL
Sassafras oil is an aromatic oil obtained from the sassafras tree. It is a flavoring agent used to make hard candies. It is also a preservative and has mild antiseptic properties. It can be used, along with other agents, for treatment of diseases of the nose and throat.

Sassafras oil is used to make pleasant-smelling solutions for bathing the horse.

SCARLET OIL
Scarlet oil is not a specific product. Rather, it is a combination of substances mixed together and dyed with *Biebrich scarlet red*, a chemical dye that gives it the characteristic color. Scarlet oil is an over-the-counter preparation for treatment of wounds (see Wound Treatments, p. 196).

Substances contained in various scarlet oil preparations include mineral oil, isopropyl alcohol, pine oil, benzyl alcohol, eucalyptus oil, methyl salicylate, and phenol (see Mineral Oil, p. 134, Isopropyl Alchohol, p. 179, Pine Oil, p. 153, Benzyl Alcohol, p. 50, Eucalyptus Oil, p. 95, Methyl Salicylate, p. 130, and Phenol, p. 150). The application of scarlet oil is recommended by some veterinarians to help promote the growth of granulation tissue. The ingredients in the mixture would seem to have little actual benefit in wound treatment.

SEDIVET® (see Romifidine Hydrochloride)

SELENIUM
Selenium is a *trace mineral* that, among other things, functions as an antioxidant in the body. Antioxidant compounds prevent or delay the deterioration of substances when they are exposed to oxygen (see Antioxidant, p. 42).

Selenium activity is apparently most important for normal muscle function. In the horse's body, it works in close association with vitamin E.

Selenium is commonly combined with vitamin E in preparations advocated for treatment of *exertional rhabdomyolysis* (*myositis* or "tying up"). Exactly what effect this combination of vitamin and mineral is supposed to have on this condition is unclear. Experimental evidence for the effectiveness of this combination at preventing rhabdomyolysis is lacking. In fact, many horses that have been previously diagnosed as tying up appear to have problems with carbohydrate metabolism, which would not be responsive to selenium supplementation.

Selenium deficiencies are reported to occur in areas where the soil is lacking in selenium, particularly in some areas of the Great Lakes region and the Eastern, Gulf and Northwestern coasts. Selenium deficiency is commonly referred to as "white muscle disease." It occurs mostly in young foals whose mothers have received inadequate levels of the mineral. Affected foals display marked muscle weakness and listlessness.

Selenium toxicity is also seen, primarily in areas such as the Rocky Mountains or Great Plains, where selenium levels in the ground are high. Plants can accumulate high levels of selenium in these areas. Signs of toxicity include lameness that is often confused with laminitis, rough and brittle hair coat and swelling of the coronary band.

SERPACIL® (see Reserpine)

SHARK CARTILAGE
Shark cartilage supplements are another bucket of water in a seemingly unending stream of products that are purportedly beneficial for the treatment of arthritis. There are no studies on the use of

shark cartilage in horses. It is likely that shark cartilage, like all cartilage, has high levels of glycosaminoglycans. *If* this is so, and *if* they are absorbed by the horse's large intestines, the theoretical benefits might be similar to those obtained with similar products (see Chondroitin Sulfate, p. 65, Perna Canaliculus, p. 149, and Polysulfated Glycosaminoglycan, p. 155). (Note the frequent use of the word "if" in this paragraph.)

Comments
There is no question that the use of such products is detrimental to sharks.

SILVER SULFADIAZINE (Silvadene®)

Silver sulfadiazine (sul-fa-DYE-a-zeen), a sulfa medicine, is a cream that is used to prevent and treat bacterial or fungal infection of the skin in people. It works by killing the fungus or bacteria. The cream is also applied to burns to prevent and treat the bacterial or fungal infection that may occur after burn injury.

Silver sulfadiazine cream is occasionally prescribed as a topical wound dressing in horses (see Wound Treatments, p. 196). It has also been applied to the eye for the treatment of fungal infections of the cornea. Its silver color is fetching.

Comments
A bacteriologist in a surgical unit combined two known antibacterial agents for burns—silver nitrate and sulfadiazine—to make the compound silver sulfadiazine. The product was first licensed in 1969 and first employed on a large scale during the Vietnam War.

SMECTITE (Biosponge®)

Dioctahedral smectite (smectite), a type of natural clay found in the ground, is commonly used to treat acute infectious diarrhea in people in many countries. There is some evidence that smectite may be helpful in reducing the duration of diarrhea when accompanied by appropriate rehydration therapy in treating acute gastroenteritis and diarrhea in children. Unfortunately, most of the human studies have important limitations that call for caution in evaluating their results. The clay is said to provide an intestinal barrier and also may absorb bacterial toxins in the intestines.

In horses, one test tube study showed that smectite bound to certain bacterial toxins, even though it had no effect on bacterial growth. However, the study also concluded that studies in live horses would be necessary to determine whether smectite might be a useful adjunctive treatment of *bacterial colitis* and *endotoxaemia* in horses. Fortunately, such conditions are not common.

There is no indication that smectite is effective for any noninfectious cause of diarrhea.

SODIUM BICARBONATE (Bicarbonate of Soda)

Sodium bicarbonate ("baking soda") is available as a white powder for oral administration or in sterile solution for intravenous (IV) administration for the horse. It has two main uses.

In solution, sodium bicarbonate may be used by some veterinarians for the treatment of *systemic acidosis* in the horse. Such conditions may occur during various types of shock. Sodium bicarbonate is sometimes given to horses with *hyperkalemic periodic paralysis (HYPP)* during an episode in an effort to reduce the amount of potassium in the blood.

Oral solutions of sodium bicarbonate ("milkshakes") have been given to horses prior to exercise in an effort to help their blood remove acid produced during exercise. This would theoretically increase endurance and performance, particularly in racing animals. This treatment can be dangerous. Not only that, but bicarbonate has been shown to be largely ineffective in increasing endurance or performance in experimental situations in racehorses. This so-called "jugging" with bicarbonate solutions is prohibited by many racing organizations.

The use of sodium bicarbonate "milkshakes" in endurance horses is *absolutely* harmful. Sweating endurance horses actually tend to become less acidic (*alkalosis*) as they exercise. Giving these horses bicarbonate before exercise would tend to make their metabolic problems worse.

Sodium bicarbonate is sometimes fed to the horse in efforts to prevent *exertional rhabdomyolysis (myositis* or "tying up"). There is one clinical report in veterinary literature of this treatment being effective in a mare that tied up frequently. However, horses may choose not to eat large amounts of sodium bicarbonate.

SODIUM BORATE

Sodium borate has some usefulness as an anti-itch agent when it is applied to the skin. It is used to help make various preparations of cosmetic ointments and lotions. Dilute sodium borate solutions have been used to make a rinse for the eye. Sodium borate has very limited therapeutic properties.

Sodium borate is a component of a hoof dressing and a coolant gel used on the horse's leg (see Hoof Dressings, p. 111, and Coolant Gel, p. 69). Its purpose in these preparations is not apparent.

SODIUM PROPIONATE (Blu-Kote®)

Sodium propionate is a *mold inhibitor* that's typically used in bakery products. It comes as a white powder. Propionates prevent microbes from producing the energy they need.

Sodium propionate is an ingredient in an over-the-counter spray sold for the treatment of wounds (see Wound Treatments, p. 196).

SORBITOL

Sorbitol is an alcohol that is most commonly used as a flavoring agent. It tastes sweet. Sorbitol has some mild effects as a laxative and moisturizer; it is found in an over-the-counter preparation for coughing in the horse. It has no known effects against coughing.

SPEARMINT OIL

Spearmint oil is derived from the spearmint plant. It is an aromatic oil that is used as a flavoring agent. It is also used in the manufacture of an over-the-counter "brace" (see Brace, p. 55). Spearmint oil has no known therapeutic value—but it smells great.

STANOZOLOL

Stanozolol (stan-OZ-a-lol) is an anabolic steroid for use as an aid in treating debilitated horses. The drug is used in an effort to promote appetite, weight gain and the general physical condition of the horse and to help speed up recovery from disease. It comes as a sterile suspension for intramuscular (IM) administration in the horse. The product must be obtained from licensed compounding pharmacies, as the commercial product (Winstrol-V®) has been removed from the market.

Precautions

Anabolic steroids have the potential to cause stallion-like behavior in the horse. These effects are reported to be lower in horses receiving stanozolol than in those receiving other similar drugs (see Boldenone Undecylenate, p. 53). The longer that a horse is kept on the drug and the higher the dosage, the more likely this complication is to be seen.

There is no data on the effects of stanozolol on stallions, pregnant mares or fetuses. The effects of other steroids have been studied in mares and it has been determined that they interrupt normal reproductive function, although normal reproductive function does eventually return once the drug is withdrawn. However, depending on the dose, normal reproductive function may take many months, or even years, to return. For that reason, use of stanozolol in mares intended for breeding should probably be avoided.

Side Effects

Because stanozolol causes retention of water and sodium, care should be used in giving this drug to horses with heart or kidney problems (see Anabolic Steroid, p. 39).

STEARIC ACID

Stearic acid is a solidifying agent used in the preparation of many creams and ointments. There are many compounds that are derived from stearic acid; the letters "S-T-E-A-R" in the chemical name of an ingredient denote its presence in a product. All stearic acid compounds are used for the same thing—as an ointment base.

In horses, stearic acid and its various derivatives are used frequently in preparing hoof dressings (see Hoof Dressings, p. 111).

STEM CELLS

Stem cell therapy is a recent addition to the treatment options for a variety of equine problems, including tendon and ligament injury and osteoarthritis. Stem cells are naturally occurring cells in the horse that can, at least theoretically, transform into a specific type of cell (e.g., bone, heart, tendon or ligament). The hope is that these cells, when injected into injured or diseased tissue, will induce better quality, or more rapid, healing.

A process is commercially available whereby stem cells are concentrated from *adipose tissue* (fat) obtained in a minor surgical procedure performed by a veterinarian. In a more invasive procedure, some veterinarians have also obtained bone marrow from the injured horse. The cells obtained from either fat or bone marrow are then implanted into the site of injury. Both products have been injected into injured tendons and ligaments, and proponents of both therapies have claimed success.

Importantly, the claims made for stem cell therapy have not yet been thoroughly, or independently, evaluated. There is currently limited information to suggest that stem cell treated horses actually do better, or heal more quickly, than horses not treated with stem cells.

Precautions
Make sure you thoroughly understand the costs and possible benefits involved before embarking down this line of treatment.

STEROID
Steroid is a term that refers to a chemical configuration that is shared by all drugs of this class. In common usage, the term has become almost meaningless and is frequently used in a negative manner because of widespread abuses of these types of drugs, as well as their considerable side effects.

A number of drugs are considered steroids. These include: (1) anabolic steroids (see Anabolic Steroid, p. 39); (2) anti-inflammatory agents (see Corticosteroid, p. 71); and (3) progesterone and other female sex hormones (see Progesterone, p. 159).

STRONGID® (see Pyrantel)

SUCRALFATE (Carafate®)
Sucralfate is a complex *polysaccharide* (sugar) that is used in the treatment of stomach and colon ulcers in the horse. It comes as a tablet for oral administration.

As sucralfate dissolves, the sugars are supposed to form a protective coating over an ulcer. Healing of the ulcer is supposed to proceed under this coating. There is scant evidence that this actually happens in horses, but the product is not harmful and finds widespread use.

SULFA

Sulfa is a general term for a group of antibacterial agents with wide use in medicine. The most commonly used sulfa drugs in the horse are sulfamethoxazole and sulfadiazine. The drugs are frequently combined with trimethoprim to increase their effectiveness (see below).

Sulfa drugs are commonly given orally but are also used topically for treatments of wounds and infection (see Wound Treatments, p. 196). Intravenous (IV) preparations of sulfa are also used by some veterinarians. An intravenous preparation of sulfadiazine and trimethoprim was previously available, but it was withdrawn because of numerous reports of adverse reactions.

SULFAMETHOXAZOLE-TRIMETHOPRIM (SMZ-TMP)

Sulfamethoxazole-trimethoprim (sul-fa-meth-OX-a-zol-tri-METH-o-prim), or SMZ-TMP (Bactrim™), is an antibacterial combination used in the treatment of a variety of infectious conditions in the horse. SMZ- TMP comes in pill form for oral administration.

Combining the two drugs increases (potentiates) the effectiveness of each drug. Because the combination of drugs is relatively inexpensive and given orally, it is popularly used in the treatment of many different types of infection in the horse.

Precautions

SMZ-TMP should theoretically not be used in horses that have *exercise-induced pulmonary hemorrhage* (known as "bleeders"). The drugs can potentially increase bleeding during exercise. The drug should be used with care in immature foals.

Side Effects

Allergic reactions to SMZ-TMP are reported in other species but are apparently rare in the horse.

SULFUR

Sulfur is one of the basic elements in nature. It is needed in extremely small amounts in the horse's diet. Neither deficiencies nor toxicities of sulfur have ever been reported in the horse. Sulfur-containing supplements available for horses include methionine and methylsulfonylmethane (see Methionine, p. 129, and Methylsulfonylmethane, p. 132).

Sulfur is also a component of various ointments, creams, shampoos and powders applied to the skin of the horse. Here, sulfur is used because it kills bacteria, kills fungus and helps remove surface skin cells.

SULFURIC ACID
Sulfuric acid is a caustic chemical that is used in various industrial processes, such as etching metal. It has no known pharmaceutical value.

Sulfuric acid is a component of an over-the-counter wound dressing available for horses (see Wound Treatments, p. 196). Sulfuric acid is not something that would normally be considered "good" for a wound.

SUPEROXIDE DISMUTASE
Superoxide dismutase is one of a group of antioxidant substances that are supposed to scavenge (pick up and remove) *free oxygen radicals*. Free oxygen radicals are byproducts of the process of inflammation. They can cause severe tissue damage. Obviously, something that could remove these radicals from the system would be of great benefit. Whether this can be effectively done or not is an open question (see Antioxidant, p. 42).

Superoxide dismutase preparations have been advertised for oral administration in the horse. Their effectiveness is unknown, however, and no studies are available to support the beneficial claims made for these products. In fact, it's unlikely that superoxide dismutase, a protein, can make it through the digestive process intact.

SWEAT WRAP
The term "sweat wrap" describes a method of applying something to the horse's limb. A medication is placed on the limb and then covered with a plastic wrap; then the leg is bandaged. The lack of air to the leg causes it to build up heat and "sweat."

After "sweating" the leg, moisture will accumulate on the leg. After the wrap is removed, frequently the skin will appear to be "tighter." Sweat wraps do not "drive" medication through the layers of the skin; that isn't possible.

The effectiveness of sweat wraps appears to be directly related to how serious the underlying problem is. They do seem to be able to help reduce minor accumulations of fluid that occur under the skin of the horse's limb. Whether this has anything to do with the sweat wrap, or just the simple act of bandaging, is not clear. They do not seem to be effective at treating injuries of deeper structures.

A number of medications are used to formulate sweat wraps, including nitrofurazone, ointment, glycerin, DMSO and corticosteroids (see Nitrofurazone, p. 140, Glycerin, p. 108, Dimethyl Sulfoxide, p. 84, and Corticosteroids, p. 71).

T

TAGAMET® (see Cimetidine)

TANNIC ACID

Tannic acid is an astringent agent, produced from various species of oak tree (see Astringent, p. 45).

Tannic acid was a compound that found much use in medicine in the past. When taken internally, it was used as a treatment for diarrhea. Applied externally, tannic acid was used as a treatment for burns. When applied to burns, tannic acid causes a hard covering to form by virtue of its astringent action. It fell out of favor as a burn treatment when it was found that tannic acid did not kill bacteria and actually promoted the death of healthy tissue—effects that are obviously undesirable. Tannic acid has also been used for the treatment of bedsores in humans.

Tannic acid is a component of an over-the-counter preparation sold for the treatment of wounds in the horse (see Wound Treatments, p. 196). Its caustic effects would seem to make it a poor choice for treatment of wounds.

TBZ (Thiabendazole, see Benzimidazole)

TEA TREE OIL

Applied to the skin, tea tree oil is commonly used for skin and skin surface infection. It may also be used as a mild antiseptic (see Antiseptic, p. 43).

Tea tree oil is obtained by the distillation of the leaves of the tea tree. It contains more than 100 compounds. Tea tree oil appears to disrupt bacterial cell membranes, which causes them to be unable to control their fluid balance (they lose their osmotic control).

Side Effects
If it's taken orally, tea tree oil and other essential oils can cause significant toxicity. In people, side effects from oral ingestion include confusion, inability to walk, disorientation and loss of coordination. In dogs and cats, the typical signs observed are depression, weakness, incoordination and muscle tremors. Such signs usually resolve in a few days. Systemic toxicities have not been reported in horses. When applied to the skin, tea tree oil can cause local irritation and inflammation, allergic skin reactions, skin dryness, and sometimes even itching, stinging, or burning.

Comments
The tea tree was named by eighteenth century sailors who made an aromatic tea from the leaves of the tree growing on the swampy southeast Australian coast.

TELMIN® (Mebendazole; see Benzimidazole)

TERBUTALINE (Brethine®)
Terbutaline (ter-BUE-ta-line) is a *bronchodilator* that is used in people to help open air passages and ease air flow in chronic lung disease. The drug has been tried in horses; however, it has not proven effective because of its poor availability and rapid clearance from the horse's bloodstream.

TESTOSTERONE
Testosterone is the hormone primarily responsible for making males be, well, males. Preparations of the hormone are occasionally used to enhance libido in slow stallions, or in an effort to make individual animals act more stallion-like.

TETRACYCLINE (Oxytetracycline, LA-200®, Bio-Mycin®, Terramycin®, Oxyject 100®, Medamycin®)
Tetracyclines are a group of antibiotics that work by interfering with

the ability of multiplying bacteria to make proteins, thereby inhibiting their growth. Tetracyclines kill a wide variety of bacteria and are employed for the treatment of many equine diseases. Oxytetracycline, the most widely used form of tetracycline, is supplied as a sterile liquid for intravenous (IV) or intramuscular (IM) administration in the horse. The IM route is not commonly used, however, because it tends to make horses' muscles sore at the site of injection.

Tetracyclines are the drugs of choice for certain parasitic infections, such as *Potomac Horse Fever (equine monocytic ehrlichiosis)*, a disease characterized by fever, depression and diarrhea.

Tetracyclines are also administered to foals with tendon contractures early in life. Some foals will be observed to develop limb deformities characterized by "knuckling over" at the fetlock joint or standing on the toes. Tetracycline is used for its ability to bind calcium; this causes muscle and tendon relaxation. After large doses of tetracyclines, contracted tendons are frequently observed to relax in affected foals.

Tetracyclines are also available in ophthalmic preparations that are sold over-the-counter for the treatment of eye infections.

Precautions
When given intravenously, rapid administration of tetracycline has caused animals to collapse. This is because it rapidly binds up body calcium, which is needed for normal muscle function, including heart muscle activity. This same effect is not seen when the drug is given slowly.

Side Effects
Tetracycline is relatively nontoxic. Some veterinarians are reluctant to use tetracycline in the horse, however, because of a report in 1973 that the drug caused *colitis* (inflammation of the colon) and severe diarrhea in the horse. As the use of the drug has become more widespread recently, especially for the treatment of Potomac Horse Fever and tendon contractures, this complication has not commonly been reported. Tetracycline appears to be much safer for horses than was previously thought.

THIAMINE (see Vitamin B₁)

THYME

Thyme is a cooking herb. In people, it has some internal applications in herbal medicine for things such as asthma and headache, although there is no evidence that it is an effective treatment. Its external use is not reported. Thyme is found in a liniment preparation sold over-the-counter for horses (see Liniment, p. 126). It is presumably a flavoring agent in this preparation. It is also included in some herbal preparations fed to horses.

THYMOL

Thymol is obtained from a plant oil by distillation. In horses, thymol is used in liniment preparations (see Liniment, p. 126). It has some use as an antibacterial and antifungal agent; however, there are many more effective agents. It has a thymelike odor that is not unpleasant, which may also be one of the reasons that it is added to horse preparations.

THYROID HORMONE (L-Thyroxine, Thyro-L®)

Disease of the thyroid gland is relatively common in humans and dogs. Affected individuals may show a number of vague clinical signs, including obesity, lethargy and intolerance to cold temperature.

A number of problems have been attributed to poor thyroid gland function in horses, including laminitis, obesity and infertility in mares. However, it's not at all clear that *hypothyroidism* (lack of normal thyroid gland function) is a real problem in horses. In fact, in experimental situations where horses have had their thyroid glands removed (totally eliminating the production of thyroid hormone), horses may become unthrifty and thin (not fat), but they don't seem to suffer any other adverse effects, such as laminitis. Mares can even reproduce normally without thyroid glands.

It is difficult to make an accurate assessment of equine thyroid gland function. Single blood tests are not necessarily accurate reflections of the horse's thyroid status; levels vary considerably during a twenty-four-hour period. In addition, other factors, including the administration of drugs and systemic disease, affect the blood levels of thyroid hormones, and may falsely affect the results of blood tests.

Nevertheless, thyroid supplementation appears to be relatively popular in horses. Thyroid hormone increases the metabolism—

when treating horses that have laminitis, it's apparently hoped that by increasing the metabolic rate, the horses will lose weight more quickly. While this may or may not occur, the best thing is to use proper diet and exercise as a means for weight control in order to keep the horse from developing problems in the first place.

There is also some indication that thyroid hormone can help decrease blood lipid concentrations, improve sensitivity to insulin and increase insulin disposal in horses. As such, thyroid hormones may have potential as a treatment for horses with reduced insulin sensitivity.

Although it is commonly done, there is good evidence to indicate that there is no reason to provide pregnant mares with thyroid hormone. Poor thyroid function is uncommon in mares and poor thyroid function is not a common cause of infertility. Thus, the practice of indiscriminately treating broodmares with thyroid hormone to enhance fertility appears questionable, at best.

TILUDRONATE (TILDREN®)

Tiludronate (tie-LOO-drone-ate) is a member of a class of drugs known as *bisphosphonates*. These drugs bind to active bone cells called *osteoclasts*. Normally, bone is an active tissue, and new bone is constantly being made and replaced. Osteoclasts help remove bone. By binding to osteoclasts, tiludronate favors bone production instead of bone removal. So, bisphosphonates find wide application in human medicine for the treatment of conditions such as osteoporosis.

In Europe, tilduronate is available in a preparation for intramuscular (IM) adminstration in horses, and the drug has been imported for use in horses in the United States. It has been used to treat horses where increased bone activity is suspected, such as *suspensory ligament disease*, inflammation of the bone of the hoof and disease of the navicular bone. There is one study that supports its use for the treatment of disease of the navicular bone.

In the United States, tiludronate is not yet approved by the US Food and Drug Administration (USFDA); however, it can be imported from Europe by a licensed veterinarian. Before the drug can meet with USFDA approval for use in horses, tiludronate, as well as other drugs of this class, will need to be studied more to demonstrate its usefulness.

TORBUGESIC® (see Butorphanol)

TRACE MINERALS

Trace minerals are inorganic (non-carbon containing) substances that are required in very small amounts (hence the term "trace") by the horse's body. They exist in interrelationships that are very complex and poorly understood. Many trace minerals are of biological importance to the animal. As a practical matter, such small amounts of these minerals are necessary that it is virtually impossible to create a diet that is lacking in them. Even when deficiencies exist, sometimes there are no clinical signs to demonstrate that fact. Some of these elements (for example, aluminum) can be demonstrated to exist in horse tissue but have no known function.

While undoubtedly important in some manner to the body, conditions where specific deficiencies of trace minerals exist are unknown in the horse. Conversely, conditions where toxicities occur as a result of oversupplementation are not reported either.

TRANEXAMIC ACID (Cyclokapron®)

In people, tranexamic acid is used for short-term control of bleeding in dental extraction procedures, after surgery or injury, for recurrent nosebleeds or in other conditions where bleeding control is required. It works by helping to prevent the breakdown of blood clots.

In horses, tranexamic acid has found some use in attempts to prevent the bleeding that occurs in the lungs of heavily exercising horses (*exercise-induced pulmonary hemorrhage*, or "bleeders").

There is no scientific proof of the efficacy or safety of tranexamic acid, and there would seem to be little justification for its race-day use.

TRANSFER FACTOR

Transfer Factor is a product being sold by a multi-level marketing approach, for a variety of conditions. It is a product which has no proven value in any illness. Claims of it "boosting the immune system" are not supported by any good research.

TRIAMCINOLONE (Vetalog®)

Triamcinolone (tri-am-SIN-o-lone) is a corticosteroid anti-inflammatory agent used in the horse (see Corticosteroid, p. 71). It is considered a long-lasting corticosteroid.

A variety of preparations of triamcinolone are available for the horse. It comes as a powder for oral administration or as a liquid for intramuscular (IM), intravenous (IV), intra-articular or intralesional administration. It also makes up a number of products that are applied to the skin, either directly or in combination with other drugs (see Panalog®, p. 144).

Precautions
Routine procedures for cleanliness should be followed to help decrease the chances of joint infection. Transient inflammatory reactions ("joint flare") may be seen after injection into joints. This will usually subside in 24 to 48 hours but must be distinguished from joint infection.

Side Effects
The systemic use of corticosteroid agents such as triamcinolone is reported to occasionally cause laminitis in some horses, although such an effect has not been reproduced in experimental settings. The reason for this side effect is unknown, although it may relate to the effect that corticosteroids have on blood vessels running to the feet. Longer-acting agents, such as triamcinolone, are considered to be more likely to cause this effect than are shorter-acting corticosteroids.

TRILOSTANE
In Europe, trilostane (TRY-low-stane) is sometimes used in the treatment of Cushing's syndrome in people. It is normally used in short-term treatment until permanent therapy is possible. In human Cushing's syndrome, the adrenal gland overproduces steroids. Although steroids are important for various functions of the body, too much can cause problems. Trilostane reduces the amount of steroids produced by the adrenal gland.

Trilostane was withdrawn from the US market in April 1994; however, it is being studied for use in dogs and horses with *Cushing's Disease* (although the name, Cushing's Disease, is the same, it is a different problem in horses than it is in dogs) because increased levels of steroids appear to be a problem both species. Further study in horses is required before the drug achieves wide use.

TRIPELENNAMINE (see Antihistamine)

TRYPTOPHAN (L-Tryptophan)

Tryptophan is an amino acid that has been promoted as a "natural" tranquilizing agent (see Amino Acid, p. 37). Tryptophan is found in high levels in many foods.

Tryptophan is a chemical needed by the horse's body to form the neurotransmitter *serotonin. Neurotransmitters* are chemicals that carry signals in the horse's nervous system. In people, high levels of serotonin are found in the fluid around the brain during sleep. Giving high levels of tryptophan is supposed to cause high levels of serotonin and make horses feel "sleepy." This effect may be desired in some show horses.

Unfortunately, there are no studies to show that tryptophan has any effect on the horse. Anecdotal reports of its effectiveness vary from "great" to "worthless."

Precautions

In humans, in the 1990s, tryptophan ingestion, even in fairly small amounts, was associated with a blood disease called eosinophil-iamyalgia. Thus, tryptophan supplements have been pulled from the human market. This condition has not as yet been reported in horses receiving this amino acid.

Comments

The "L" in L-tryptophan is a chemistry term that refers to its chemical configuration.

TURPENTINE

Turpentine is a light oil that is obtained from processing crude oil. Purified turpentine was used as a diuretic and antiparasitic agent in people many, many years ago. Newer and safer drugs have long since replaced the use of turpentine as a pharmaceutical.

In horses, turpentine is used primarily on the hoof and is a component of a variety of hoof dressings (see Hoof Dressings, p. 111). It also is reported to be a toughening agent for the hoof, especially the sole.

There is an over-the-counter wound preparation that contains turpentine (see Wound Treatments, p. 196). What possible benefit could be obtained from putting turpentine on delicate, healing tissue escapes understanding.

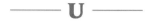

U

ULCERGARD® (see Omeprazole)

UREA
Urea is a nitrogen-containing compound that is found in urine. At one time, it was used as an oral diuretic in humans, but it is only used intravenously (IV) today.

Urea is a component of an over-the-counter dressing used on horse hooves (see Hoof Dressings, p. 111). What purpose it might serve is unknown.

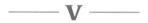

V

VALERIAN ROOT
Valerian products are made from the root of a tall, wispy plant, which is grown to decorate gardens but also grows wild in damp grasslands. Its umbrella-like heads top grooved, erect and hollow stems. Its dark green leaves are pointed at the tip and hairy underneath. Small, sweet-smelling white, light purple or pink flowers bloom in early summer.

Valerian is native to the Americas, Asia and Europe. The plant became particularly popular in Europe starting in the seventeenth century and has been used for insomnia, anxiety and restlessness. It's most well-researched use is as a calming or tranquilizing agent to help people sleep.

Precautions
Products containing valerian root can result in testing positive for forbidden substances in the blood or urine of a horse. The United States Equestrian Federation (USEF) recommends that a horse be withdrawn from competition for at least seven days after injestion of any product containing valerian root.

VALIUM® (see Diazepam)

VASELINE® (see Petrolatum)

VENICE TURPENTINE (see Turpentine)

VERVAIN (Common Verbena)

Like many herbal products, the uses of vervain are innumerable. In people, it is used for sore throats and other oral and pharyngeal inflammation and has been applied topically for the treatment of wounds. It also is a flavoring agent in alcoholic beverages, and adds fragrance to some soaps.

Some preliminary research suggests that vervain might have some weak antimicrobial activity. There is no scientific information to suggest that vervain has any therapeutic application in horses.

VETALOG® (see Triamcinolone)

VITAMIN

Vitamin is a general term that is used to describe a variety of unrelated organic compounds that occur in most foods in small amounts. They are necessary for the normal metabolic functions of the body. With the exception of vitamin E, vitamin deficiencies are not known to exist naturally in the horse. Normally, the horse's body provides all of its own vitamins (unlike humans), by synthesis from its own system, by exposure to sunlight, and by absorption of vitamins produced by the bacteria that live in the gastrointestinal tract.

There appears to be little need for vitamin supplementation in the horse according to most studies. However, most vitamins are available in relatively inexpensive forms and they are widely used. The rule for feeding and supplementing horses seems to be: "When in doubt, use vitamins." Fortunately, considering the frequency with which they are given, vitamins are safe supplements to give to horses and are only toxic in large doses.

VITAMIN A

Vitamin A maintains the normal structure and function of the *epithelial cells*, the surface cells that occur throughout the body. It is also needed for normal bone growth, has a well-defined role in maintaining normal vision, and is needed for normal reproductive function in both males and females.

Deficiencies of vitamin A first show up as changes in the epithelial surfaces. Surfaces become dryer and less resilient; their mucus-secreting capacity becomes reduced. As epithelial surfaces lose their normal capabilities, the potential for infection increases. "Night blindness" and excessive tear formation are ocular signs of vitamin A deficiencies. Reproductive efficiency is also greatly reduced.

It has been said that if the feed given to a horse has the color green in it, there is sufficient vitamin A for the needs of the horse. The amount of vitamin A in feed is roughly equal to the amount of the color green in the feed. Additionally, a three- to six-month supply of vitamin A is stored in the liver of the horse.

Vitamin and mineral supplements commonly contain vitamin A. Adding vitamin A supplements to mineral mixtures rapidly destroys the vitamin.

Precautions
Vitamin A is one of the few vitamins that can cause toxicities. Fortunately, the dosages required for toxicities are quite large. The signs of toxicities are similar to those of deficiencies (see above).

VITAMIN B
The B-vitamins are a whole group of vitamins with a variety of metabolic functions in the horse. They are found in plentiful supply in horse feed. The microorganisms of the horse's digestive tract also manufacture B-vitamins in large amounts. In normal horses, these two sources provide more than enough of the B-vitamins needed to meet the horse's requirements.

B-vitamins are among the most commonly supplemented vitamins in the horse, possibly because of the fact that people do not get B-vitamins from the bacteria in their intestines and sometimes dietary sources are inadequate (in some vegetarian diets, for example). Hence, B-vitamin deficiencies are occasionally seen in humans. The story isn't necessarily the same for horses, however.

B-vitamins are commonly given as a supplement to horses when they are in disease states. The B-vitamins are not stored in the horse's body for long periods of time, and chronic disease or decreased food intake may be considered reasons to provide B-vitamin supplementation to a horse. It is virtually impossible (and extremely expensive) to determine that a horse might be deficient in a specific B-vitamin, and supplements are relatively cheap; hence, frequently they are given "just in case" something might be needed.

It is commonly thought that B-vitamins can serve as an appetite stimulant. Experimental evidence with B-vitamins has shown no effect in stimulating the horse's appetite.

Sterile "vitamin B-complex" solutions are available for intramuscular (IM) injection in the horse. These products typically contain vitamins B_1, B_2, B_3, B_6, pantothenic acid and B_{12}. Warnings on the label suggest caution because administration of vitamin B_1 has resulted in *anaphylactic* (allergic) shock in some animals.

VITAMIN B₁ (Thiamine)

Vitamin B_1 (thiamine) is important in the production of energy by the cells of the horse's body. It is present in high levels in plant products, like hay. Interestingly, it is easily destroyed by heat and cooking, so thiamine may have to be added back to heat-processed feeds to restore preprocessing levels. Intestinal bacteria produce a great deal of thiamine. It is impossible to give a horse a normal diet that is thiamine-deficient. Dietary thiamine deficiencies have only been seen in horses with experimentally produced diets.

Deficiencies of thiamine have been associated with the ingestion of plants that produce enzymes that break down thiamine or have anti-thiamine activity. Signs of thiamine deficiency include loss of appetite, weight loss, hemorrhage of the gums and heart-rate abnormalities.

Thiamine toxicity is very unlikely if the vitamin is given orally. A dose of 1000 times that which is recommended appears to be safe. High doses of thiamine have been injected into the horse in an effort to provide "natural" tranquilization. Indeed, some work done in Australia suggested that horses given thiamine seemed to be less excitable while walking to the racetrack. However, other studies have been unable to repeat this effect.

Side Effects

A negative side effect of thiamine is reported to be anaphylactic (allergic) shock. This effect may be seen more often when the vitamin is given intravenously (IV). Excessive blood levels of thiamine are prohibited by racing associations and the United States Equestrian Federation (USEF).

VITAMIN B$_2$ (Riboflavin)

Vitamin B$_2$ (riboflavin), another vitamin important for normal metabolic activity in the horse, is also provided in high levels in horse feed and produced by the bacteria of the horse's intestines. Neither deficiencies nor toxicities of vitamin B$_2$ have ever been reported in the horse.

VITAMIN B$_3$ (Niacin)

Vitamin B$_3$ (niacin) is important for energy production in all cells of the horse's body. As with all B-vitamins, the horse's normal intake and intestinal production appear to provide vast amounts of vitamin B$_3$ for the horse. Niacin can also be manufactured from the amino acid tryptophan in the horse's tissues (see Tryptophan, p. 187). Specific deficiencies or toxicities have not been reported in the horse.

VITAMIN B$_6$

Vitamin B$_6$ is actually a generic term for three similar compounds that have equal vitamin activity: *pyridoxal, pyridoxine* and *pyridoxamine*. No dietary requirements for these have been established in the horse and their precise functions are not known. Ample levels are provided from the normal sources in the horse. Deficiencies or toxicities of vitamin B$_6$ are unknown.

VITAMIN B$_{12}$ (Cyanocobalamin)

Vitamin B$_{12}$ (cyanocobalamin) is the only B-vitamin that is not found in large amounts in the horse's feed. However, synthesis of vitamin B$_{12}$ by the intestinal bacteria of the horse is more than adequate to meet the horse's needs, even when extremely low amounts of the vitamin are supplied in the diet. Cyanocobalamin is needed for red blood cells to mature.

Vitamin B$_{12}$ is available as a sterile solution for intramuscular (IM) or intravenous (IV) injection at a variety of concentrations. It is commonly used in an effort to "pep up" or "build blood" in horses, but there has been no observed response to vitamin B$_{12}$ injections in experimental situations. Injected B$_{12}$ is removed rapidly from the blood by the kidney and liver.

There are no reports of deficiencies or toxicities in the horse.

VITAMIN C (Ascorbic Acid)

Also known as ascorbic acid, vitamin C is found in high levels in many vegetable compounds (like hay). It has a variety of important metabolic functions. Like vitamin E and the trace mineral selenium, vitamin C is also an antioxidant (see Vitamin E, below, Selenium, p. 172, and Antioxidant, p. 42).

Although sometimes recommended for treatment of various conditions, especially arthritis, Vitamin C deficiencies are unknown in horses because horses synthesize it in their bodies. In humans, a deficiency of vitamin C causes scurvy, a condition characterized by weakness, anemia, spongy gums and a tendency toward bruising and bleeding.

Supplemental vitamin C has no known beneficial effects in the horse.

VITAMIN D

Vitamin D is formed in the tissues of the horse by the action of the sun's rays on a by-product of the body's cholesterol. Because vitamin D levels are related to exposure to the sun, it is very difficult to make a horse deficient in vitamin D.

Vitamin D is stored in all tissues of the horse's body. It helps to maintain calcium and phosphorus levels in the body. Calcium and phosphorus are two minerals that are needed for bone formation (see Calcium, p. 57, and Phosphorus, p. 152). Accordingly, vitamin D deficiencies, on the rare occasions that they are seen, occur in growing animals and show up as abnormalities of bone formation (*rickets*).

Vitamin D toxicity has been reported in horses. Most commonly it is associated with eating the wild jasmine plant (*Cestrum diurnum*), although there are reports of horses being given too much vitamin D in their diets. Signs of toxicity are stiffness and soreness, lack of eating, weight loss, excessive drinking, frequent urination and calcification of the kidneys. The prognosis for recovery from vitamin D toxicosis is poor.

VITAMIN E

Vitamin E is necessary in the diet of the horse for normal reproduction, muscle development, red blood cell function and a variety of other biochemical functions. It is found in high levels in cereals, fresh pasture, wheat germ oil and various grains.

Vitamin E is also an antioxidant. Antioxidant compounds prevent or delay the deterioration of substances when they are exposed to oxygen (see Antioxidant, p. 42). Because of its antioxidant properties, vitamin E is frequently administered as treatment or prevention for acute or *chronic equine exertional rhabdomyolysis*, also known as "tying up," *myositis* or *azoturia*. Theoretically, vitamin E would help prevent further degrading of muscle cells. Typically, it is combined with selenium, a trace mineral, for treatment or prevention of this condition. No scientific evidence exists to support the effectiveness of this treatment for rhabdomyolysis, and most research suggests that rhabdomyolsis is caused by other factors, many of which appear to be genetic.

Deficiencies of vitamin E cause *equine motor neuron syndrome*, a condition characterized by incoordination and muscle twitching. The condition is usually seen in horses that have inadequate access to green forage.

Vitamin E is also available in various ointments and oils for application to wounds in the horse, as well as in various hoof dressings (see Wound Treatments, p. 196, and Hoof Dressings, p. 111). There is no evidence that vitamin E has any effect in these areas. Application of vitamin E to the surface of a wound does not decrease the formation of scar tissue, nor does it increase the speed of or the amount of hair regrowth.

VITAMIN K
This group of vitamins promotes clotting of the blood by increasing the synthesis of one of the clotting factors (*prothrombin*) in the liver. High amounts of vitamin K occur in alfalfa hay. Vitamin K deficiencies are not known to occur in horses.

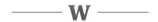

W

WHEAT GERM OIL
Wheat germ oil is a plant oil that is often seen in health food stores. It is edible and contains various vitamins and fatty acids.

Wheat germ oil is also a component of various hoof dressings for the horse (see Hoof Dressings, p. 111). It is presumably used for the same reasons as other plant oils, such as linseed or coconut oils (see Linseed Oil, p. 126, and Coconut Oil, p. 68).

WHITE LOTION

White lotion is a mild solution of zinc sulfate. It is an astringent and a very mild antibacterial agent.

Some veterinarians use white lotion to treat skin diseases of the horse.

WHITE WILLOW BARK (*Salix alba*)

In people, white willow bark and willow bark extracts are taken orally, primarily for various types of pain. The active constituent of willow bark is thought to be *salicin*. Salicin is metabolized to salicyl alcohol and then to salicylic acid. From there, metabolism is the same as aspirin, the pharmaceutical product which was ultimately synthezied from white willow bark (see Aspirin, p. 43).

There is little scientific evidence to suggest that white willow bark is effective for the purposes for which it is intended in people, and none in horses. White willow bark can be irritating to the gastrointestinal tract.

Comments

The composer, Ludwig von Beethoven, is thought to have ingested toxic amounts of salicin, which may have contributed to his death.

WINSTROL-V® (see Stanozolol, Anabolic Steroid)

WINTERGREEN OIL (see Methyl Salicylate)

WITCH HAZEL

Witch hazel is a volatile liquid distilled from a plant. It has use as a mild astringent (see Astringent, p. 45). It is also used as a mild counterirritant (see Counterirritant, p. 74).

In horses, witch hazel is used in formulating a variety of liniment and coolant-gel-type products that are sold over-the-counter (see Liniment, p. 126, and Coolant Gel, p. 69). It has a very distinctive smell but little or no therapeutic value.

WORMWOOD OIL

Wormwood extracts come from an aromatic plant. The extract is bitter and used in flavoring certain wines and making *absinthe*, a green liqueur. In the 1800s, wormwood extract was also used to treat sprains.

Wormwood oil is found in a commonly used liniment preparation sold over-the-counter for horses (see Liniment, p. 126). What effectiveness it might have is unknown.

WOUND TREATMENTS

Wounds of the horse are an unfortunate and somewhat common occurrence, since horses do seem to be accident-prone. Wounds that go deep through the skin surface and reveal or penetrate underlying structures should be treated by a veterinarian as rapidly as possible. After wounds occur, horse owners generally want to clean them with a disinfectant solution, such as chlorhexidine, povidone-iodine or hydrogen peroxide (see Chlorhexadine, p. 64, Povidone-Iodine, p. 158, and Hydrogen Peroxide, p. 115). When done by the owner, the benefits obtained from cleaning wounds are more likely related to the mechanical removal of debris than to the particular solution that is chosen to do it.

Surface scrapes—those wounds that remove hair and/or cause reddening of the skin—rarely, if ever, require treatment of any kind. Horse owners, however, frequently feel that it is necessary to apply some sort of antibacterial, antibiotic or vitamin preparation to these areas to "help" healing. In truth, it is virtually impossible to do anything to prevent rapid healing of these superficial scrapes; treatment is often more for the horse owner than for the horse! There is also no treatment available that serves to promote or speed hair growth on these superficial wounds.

After surgical repair of wounds, antibiotic *wound dressings* are frequently applied to the surface. In sutured wounds, however, a wound dressing may not be all that important. Many surgeons feel that a sutured wound doesn't need to be covered with any type of medicated dressing, as long as it is protected from additional trauma or contamination.

Finally, many different types of wound dressings are commonly applied to *granulation tissue.* Granulation tissue forms when the skin edges of a wound are too far apart to reunite with sutures, usually because of tissue loss. The appearance of granulation tissue is part of normal healing in these wounds. Horse owners, however, become greatly concerned about excessive granulation tissue, or "proud flesh."

Proud flesh describes granulation tissue that has grown beyond the surface of the wound. Once beyond the wound surface, granulation tissue can proliferate and look ugly. Proud flesh is not abnormal tissue, but normal tissue that has been allowed to overgrow. It is not bad for a wound. It is not dangerous to the horse. Its presence does not mean that a horse will become permanently disfigured. It may mean that not enough attention has been paid to the wound, since there's no reason why a wound that has been properly cared for should develop proud flesh.

It is occasionally necessary to control the growth of granulation tissue so that a wound can heal. The pressure from a properly applied bandage can help limit the growth of proud flesh. The growth of this tissue can also be controlled by the use of corticosteroid-based ointments (see Corticosteroid, p. 71). These ointments slow the growth of granulation tissue when they are applied to the surface of the tissue, but when applied starting five days from the initial injury, corticosteroid ointments do not slow down the new epithelial cells growing in from the sides of the wound. Excessive granulation tissue also can be cut back with a scalpel.

Precautions
What should not be done to granulation tissue is to apply substances that are caustic and damaging to the fresh tissue. Things like lime, kerosene, copper sulfate, sulfuric acid, pine tar or silver nitrate are awful things to put on fresh tissue (see Lime, p. 126, Copper Sulfate, p. 71, Sulfuric Acid, p. 179, and Pine Tar, p. 153). Remember, granulation tissue is normal, healing tissue. It is trying to heal your horse's wound. Don't hurt it.

If you put caustic chemicals on the tissue, you will induce a chemical burn. The body will not heal over this newly damaged tissue until the damaged tissue itself has had time to heal. When used as wound treatments, caustic agents cause a hard scab to form on tissue because they cause surface proteins to come out of the solution (this action is called *precipitation*). Although they may kill bacteria directly, the formation of a chemical scab on healing tissue is not necessarily beneficial. In fact, the growth of bacteria may even be favored by the protection of the chemically caused scab.

Comments
Wounds will try to heal in spite of the wide variety of inappropriate

and implausible (e.g., bacon grease) substances applied to them. One rule of thumb used by some surgeons is that you should never put anything on a wound that you would not put in your own eye. It's not a bad rule to follow, although you probably shouldn't test things that way.

WYAMINE SULFATE
Wyamine is a drug used in humans to increase blood pressure. In horses, some people have tried to use it as a stimulant to improve racing performance. Wyamine has not been tested on horses and its effects are unsubstantiated.

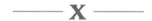

XXTERRA®
Xxterra is advertised as a "natural" treatment for various skin cancers of the horse.

Two of the primary components of the product are bloodroot and high concentrations of zinc chloride. While bloodroot has no known anti-cancer properties, high concentrations of zinc chloride are caustic, and have been used to remove such things as warts in people (see Bloodroot, p. 53, and Zinc Chloride, p. 200).

XYLAZINE HYDROCHLORIDE (Rompun®, Anased®)
Xylazine is a short-acting sedative for horses. It is also a potent analgesic, and it is very commonly used for the control of colic pain. In fact, some clinicians feel that if a horse's abdominal pain cannot be controlled by xylazine, the problem most likely will require surgery to correct. Xylazine is also a relaxant of skeletal muscle. After the drug is given to the horse, the horse's head drops within a very short time, indicating that he is sedated. Xylazine is often used in combination with other drugs when putting a horse under general anesthesia for surgery.

Xylazine comes as a sterile liquid. It can be given intravenously (IV) or intramuscularly (IM) and its effects are dose-related.

Xylazine is also used to cause chemical ejaculation in stallions that may have difficulty being collected under normal circumstances.

Precautions
In large doses, xylazine can cause a horse to become unsteady. It is particularly important to note that even when horses are sedated with large doses of xylazine, they can still react to stimuli. Horses have been observed to kick out quickly, even while sedated with relatively large doses of this drug.

Horses intended for use in shows must not have traces of xylazine in their systems.

Side Effects
After dosage with xylazine, it is common to observe a heart rhythm abnormality known as *second degree A-V (atrio-ventricular) block*. This is best described as the heart having an irregular pattern, characterized by the heart rhythm slowing down and then skipping a beat. This usually disappears within a few minutes of administration of the drug and is not a health threat to the horse. Caution in giving the drug to horses with heart problems would be advisable, however.

Xylazine relaxes the muscles of the horse. It can reduce the respiratory rate, as is seen in natural sleep. Care should be taken in using xylazine in horses with depressed respiration.

Sweating is also common after administration of xylazine. This is an effect of the drug on sweat glands and is not a sign of an abnormal or dangerous response.

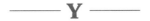

YOHIMBINE
Yohimbe is the name of an evergreen tree that is native to Zaire, Cameroon and Gabon. The bark of the yohimbe tree contains the alkaloid yohimbine, which has effects on the circulatory system. In people, yohimbine is primarily used as an aphrodisiac and for erectile dysfunction in males.

In horses, yohimbine is primarily used to reverse the effects of detomodine or xylazine, after such tranquilizers are given for various procedures (see Detomodine, p. 78, and Xylazine, p. 198).

YUCCA
Yucca is a feed supplement that is purported to be for the relief of

199

arthritic conditions of the horse. In people, it can also be applied topically for a variety of skin conditions. It is obtained from a cactus-like plant.

Most preparations are combined with anise, the seed that gives the flavoring to black licorice.

Herbal pharmacy texts give no information as to why yucca should be beneficial in the treatment of arthritis.

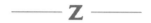

Z

ZANTAC (see Ranitidine)

ZIMECTRIN® (see Ivermectin)

ZIMECTRIN GOLD® (see Ivermectin, Praziquantel)

ZINC

Zinc is a trace mineral that is an important part of the many enzymes associated with skeletal development in the horse (see Trace Minerals, p. 185).

Zinc deficiencies have not been reported in horses. It is virtually impossible for a horse not to get enough zinc in his diet.

Zinc toxicity has been reported in horses, primarily where pastures have been contaminated from metal-smelting activity or where water has been contaminated by porous galvanized pipe. Bone and joint abnormalities have been identified in horses with zinc toxicity. Clinical signs of zinc intoxication include stiffness, lameness and joint swelling.

ZINC CHLORIDE

Zinc chloride in high concentrations is a caustic chemical and has been used to treat corns, calluses and warts in people. It is found in high concentration in a "natural" product intended to treat various skin cancers in horses (see Xxterra®, p. 198). Pastes of 20 percent zinc chloride have been used to treat the same cancers by some veterinarians, at a much lower cost than for the proprietary product.

ZINC OXIDE

Zinc oxide is a white, mildly astringent and antiseptic ointment that is sometimes used as a protectant for the horse's skin against sunlight in hot, sunny climates (see Astringent, p. 45, and Antiseptic, p. 43). It is also the essential ingredient in calamine lotion, a soothing lotion that people put on their own itchy skin.

ZINC SULFATE (see White Lotion)

BIBLIOGRAPHY

Adams, M.R., ed. *Veterinary Pharmacology and Therapeutics*. 8th ed. Ames, Iowa: Iowa State University Press, 2001.

Balch, J. F., and P. A. Balch. *Prescription for Nutritional Healing*. Garden Park City, New York: Avery Publishing Group, 1990.

Barnum, R. C. *The People's Home Library*. Toronto: Imperial Publishing Company, 1916.

Bennett, K., ed. *Compendium of Veterinary Products*. 2nd ed. Port Huron, Michigan: North American Compendiums, Inc., 1993.

Beringer, P, DerMarderosian, A, Felton, L, et al, eds. *Remington: The Science and Practice of Pharmacy*. 21st ed. Philadephia: Lippincott, Williams and Wilkins, 2006.

Budiansky, Stephen. "Don't Bet on Faster Horses." *New Scientist*. Issue 2042 (10 August 1996).

Dorland's Illustrated Medical Dictionary. 20th ed. Philadelphia: WB Saunders Company, 2000.

Editors of the UC Berkeley "Wellness Letter." *The Wellness Encyclopedia*. New York: Houghton Mifflin Company, 1991.

Foster, S, Tyler, VE. *Tyler's Honest Herbal: A Sensible Guide to the Use of Herbs and Related Remedies*. Binghamton, New York: Haworth Press, 1999.

Herbert V. "The Antioxidant Supplement Myth." *American Journal Clinical Nutrition* 60 (1994):157–8.

Hinchcliff, KW, Kaneps, AJ, Geor, RJ. *Equine Sports Medicine and Surgery*. Edinburgh, Scotland: Saunders, 2003.

Hinchcliff, K.W, and Sams, R.A., eds. "Drug Use in Performance Horses." *The Veterinary Clinics of North America, Equine Practice*. 9:3. Philadelphia: WB Saunders and Company, 1993.

Hintz, H. F., ed. "Clinical Nutrition." *The Veterinary Clinics of North America, Equine Practice.* 6:2. Philadelphia: WB Saunders and Company, 1990.

Hooper, L., Thompson, R.L., Harrison, R.A., et al. "Risks and Benefits of Omega-3 Fats for Mortality, Cardiovascular Disease, and Cancer: Systematic Review." *British Medical Journal.* 332 (7544) (2006): 752–60.

McKinnon, A. 0., and Voss, J. L. *Equine Reproduction.* Philadelphia: Lea & Febiger, 1993.

National Research Council. *Nutrient Requirements of Horses.* 5th ed. Washington, DC: National Academy Press, 1989.

http://www.naturaldatabase.com

Reed, S, Bayly, W, McEachern, R, et al. *Equine Internal Medicine.* 2nd ed. Philadelphia: Saunders, 2003.

Robbers, JE, Tyler, VE. *Tyler's Herbs of Choice:The Therapeutic Use of Phytomedicinals.* Binghamton, New York: Haworth Press, 1999.

Robinson, N.E., ed. *Current Therapy in Equine Medicine 5.* Philadelphia: WB Saunders and Company, 2003.

Shang, A, Huwiler-Muntener, K, Nartey, L, et al. "Are the Clinical Effects of Homoeopathy Placebo Effects? Comparative Study of Placebo-Controlled Trials of Homoeopathy and Allopathy. *The Lancet* 366(9487) (2005): 726–32.

White, N. A., and Moore, J. N. *Current Practice of Equine Surgery.* New York: J. B. Lippincott Company, 1990.

INDEX OF BRAND NAMES